PATHOLOGY OF THE SPINAL CORD

Pathology of the Spinal Cord

J. TREVOR HUGHES
M.A., D.Phil. (Oxford), M.D. (Manchester),
F.R.C.P. (Edinburgh), F.R.C.Path.

Consultant Neuropathologist, Radcliffe Infirmary, Oxford;
Clinical Lecturer in Neuropathology, University of Oxford

Second edition

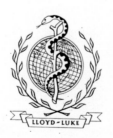

LLOYD-LUKE (MEDICAL BOOKS) LTD
49 NEWMAN STREET
LONDON
1978

FIRST EDITION 1966
SECOND EDITION . . . 1978

PRINTED IN ENGLAND BY
THE PITMAN PRESS, BATH

ISBN 0 85324 100 7

FOREWORD

THE purpose of this book is to present a comprehensive and yet concise description of the pathological changes of the spinal cord resulting from the various processes affecting the vertebral column and the spinal cord itself. The need for such a book, which covers practically the whole field of spinal cord pathology and correlates the author's wide personal experience with that of other workers in this field, has been urgently felt for some time.

In the course of his career as a pathologist, Dr. Trevor Hughes came to Stoke Mandeville Hospital in Aylesbury, where he became closely associated with the work of the National Spinal Injuries Centre and devoted much time and thought to the pathology of the spinal cord, especially following traumatic lesions. He had the good fortune to continue his studies and enlarge his experience in this complex subject of neuropathology at the Radcliffe Infirmary, Oxford, and has become an expert in this field.

For the clinician who is engaged in the management and re-habilitation of paraplegics and tetraplegics due to injuries of the spine as well as spondylosis, Dr. Hughes' own research on vascular disorders will be of particular interest. One can only hope that these chapters will be widely read and will disseminate knowledge about the hazards and dangers of hasty operative procedures in the acute stages of traumatic lesions of the vertebral column involving the spinal cord.

Apart from the author's personal experience, this book gives an excellent survey of the old and modern literature of the neuro-pathology of the spinal cord.

After reading through the pages, I warmly recommend this book as a valuable and reliable guide to all colleagues who are engaged in clinical pathology as well as research in spinal cord afflictions.

SIR LUDWIG GUTTMANN, C.B.E., M.D., F.R.C.P., F.R.C.S., F.R.S. *Director, Stoke Mandeville Sports Stadium for the Paralysed and Other Disabled.*

PREFACE TO THE SECOND EDITION

DURING the eleven years which have elapsed since the production of the first edition of this book, the subject of neuropathology has shared in the general expansion of all biological sciences. The enlargement of the subject is reflected in the extensive revision made in the majority of the chapters. However, although much new material has been added, the original object of the book has been retained—that of providing a concise textbook of diseases and traumas affecting the human spinal cord.

Oxford J. TREVOR HUGHES
June 1977

PREFACE TO THE FIRST EDITION

IN writing this monograph on the pathology of the spinal cord I had in mind the needs of two groups of readers. My first aim was to provide a concise descriptive account for the use of neurologists, neurosurgeons, and in particular those clinical practitioners who have specialised with such notable success in the care of paraplegic and quadriplegic patients. But it is hoped that the work will also be of value to a wider medical public including general physicians, and possibly paediatric and geriatric specialists. The second group of readers for whom I have striven to cater are those morbid anatomists who, although skilled in necropsy and biopsy work, find the examination of the spinal cord technically exacting and their histological preparations difficult to interpret. I judge this to be so from the frequency with which cases of this kind are submitted to me for examination. For these readers, I have included a chapter with practical advice in obtaining and handling the necropsy tissues. The spinal cord, when correctly prepared and examined, is the easiest part of the central nervous system to interpret at necropsy. I hope to convince morbid anatomists without special training in neuropathology that, with care and attention to detail, but with only minor variations of their customary techniques, they can obtain excellent results in the examination of the spinal cord.

My list of acknowledgements to those who have assisted me in this work is necessarily a long one. Mr. J. Pennybacker and Mr. J. M. Potter of the department of Neurosurgery, and Dr. W. Ritchie Russell, Dr. C. W. M. Whitty, Dr. J. M. K. Spalding, and Dr. Honor M. V. Smith of the department of Neurology regularly participate in our clinico-pathological meetings at the Radcliffe Infirmary, where many of the points dealt with in this book have been cogently discussed. I am indebted to Dr. D. B. Brownell, Mr. J. Pennybacker, Mr. J. M. Potter, Dr. Honor M. V. Smith and Dr. D. R. Oppenheimer who have all read the manuscript. I have especial reason to thank my colleague Dr. D. B. Brownell who has assisted at all stages of the preparation of the book and has compiled the index. Miss B. Newton, librarian of the postgraduate medical library of the Radcliffe Infirmary, has checked all the references and procured many journals and in this respect the staff of the Radcliffe Science Library, Oxford have also been extremely helpful. For secretarial assistance I wish to thank Miss Elisabeth Wilson and Mrs. Joan Smith who together have typed the manuscript. For many years Mr. R. Beesley and Miss Eileen Stanley have prepared innumerable spinal-cord sections which have been the foundation of the observations detailed here. For photographic assistance I am indebted to the departments of photography of Mr. E. L. Tugwell and Dr. Parry, my use of the latter being through the kindness of Dr. A. H. T. Robb-Smith, Director of Pathology, United Oxford Hospitals. I am grateful to Dr. L. Guttmann who, during my first steps in Neuropathology at Stoke Mandeville Hospital in 1956, actively encouraged my interest in the pathology of the spinal cord.

Finally I should like to record the courtesy and consideration that I have received from Mr. Douglas Luke during the publication of this book.

J. TREVOR HUGHES

October 1965

ACKNOWLEDGEMENTS

In the preparation of the second edition, I am again grateful to my clinical and neuropathological colleagues, and have drawn heavily on the resources of my laboratory technical staff, ably led by Mr. Ron Beesley. The Cairns Library of the Radcliffe Infirmary, and the Radcliffe Science Library have constantly traced obscure references and obtained rare journals. All the references cited have been checked by Mr. Ian Kennedy of the Cairns Library. For secretarial assistance I am indebted to Mrs. Joan Smith and to Mrs. Carmel Spicer. Dr. Betty Brownell has kindly revised the index that she prepared for the first edition.

Finally I am grateful again for the continued kindness and help of my publishers Lloyd-Luke in bringing the second edition to press.

I wish to make the following detailed acknowledgements for permission to reproduce illustrations:

FIGURES 1, 4, and 10, from Glees, P. and Meller, K. (1964). *Int. J. Paraplegia*, **2**, 77–95, by permission of the authors and editor; FIGS. 11, 12, and 13 from Blechschmidt, E. (1961). *The Stages of Human Development before Birth*. S. Karger, Basel/New York, by permission of the author and publisher; FIG. 15 from Perret, G. (1960). *Neurology* (*Minneap.*), **10**, 51–60, by permission of the author and editors; FIG. 17 from Potter, E. L. (1961). *Pathology of the Fetus and Infant*, 2nd edit. Year Book Medical Publishers, Chicago, by permission of the author and publisher; FIG. 23 from Adams, H. D. and Van Geertruyden, H. H. (1956). *Ann. Surg.*, **144**, 574–610, by permission of the authors and the editorial and advisory board; FIGS. 24, and 25 from Hughes, J. T. (1964). *Int. J. Paraplegia*, **2**, 2–14, by permission of the editor; FIGS. 28*a* and *b* from Hubert, J. P. *et al.* (1974). *Acta Neurol.* (*Belg.*), **74**, 297–305, by permission of the authors and the editor; FIGS. 29, 30, 31, and 32 from Hughes, J. T. (1971). *Neurology* (*Minneap.*), **21**, 794–800 by permission of the editors; FIG. 35 by courtesy of Dr. H. J. Harris and the Department of Photography, Stoke Mandeville Hospital; FIG. 36 from Bedbrook, G. M. (1963). *Int. J. Paraplegia*, **1**, 215–227 by permission of the author and the editor; FIG. 38 by courtesy of Mr. G. M. Bedbrook F.R.C.S.; FIG. 42 by courtesy of Dr. U. Rowlett and Professor P. M. Daniel; FIGS. 47a and b from Hesketh, K. T. (1965). *J. Neurol. Neurosurg. Psychiat.*, **28,** 445–448, by permission of the author and editor; FIGS. 48a and b from Herskowitz, A. (1972). *J. Neurosurg.*, **36,** 494–498, by permission of the author and editor; FIGS. 49a, b and c from Bodian, D. (1948). *Bull. Johns. Hopk. Hosp.*, **83,** 1–107, by permission of the author and the editors; FIG. 54 from Hoffmann, G. T. (1960). *J. Neurosurg.*, **17,** 327–330, by permission of the author and the editorial board; FIG. 57 by courtesy of Professor W. Krücke; FIG. 61 from Russell, D. S. and Rubinstein, L. J. (1963). *Pathology of Tumours of the Nervous System*, 2nd edit. Edward Arnold, London, by permission of the authors and the publisher; FIG. 67a by courtesy of Miss Audrey J. Arnott and Professor P. M. Daniel; FIG. 70 by courtesy of Professor P. M. Daniel; FIGS. 72, 73, and 74 by courtesy of Miss Margaret C. McLarty.

CONTENTS

CHAPTER I

INTRODUCTION

The structure of the human spinal cord is unique in many ways which are reflected in the particular features encountered in its diseases. Although of extraordinary functional diversity the component cells of the spinal cord are morphologically of few fundamental types. The neurones have their cell bodies in the grey matter and send out long axons, which form the white matter. The supporting tissue consists of the three types of glia to which may be added the few ependymal cells forming the central canal. Connective tissue is present in the form of fibroblasts with collagen or reticulin fibres. The connective tissue accompanies the vascular endothelial cells forming the blood vessels in the lumen of which are the variety of cells transported in the blood. This simplicity of component cells means that the variety of reaction permitted to the spinal cord, whether as a sequel of injury or disease, is limited. For an exhaustive treatment of the behaviour of neurones and glia the reader is referred to the larger texts listed among the references given at the end of the chapter. Of particular value are the reviews of Penfield (1932), Cajal (1952, 1959), Glees (1961), Hydén (1967), and Bourne (1968–72); and also the introductory chapters of Vol. XIII of Lubarsch *et al.* (1955–58), of *Greenfield's Neuropathology* (Blackwood *et al.*, 1976), and of Minckler (1968–72). In this chapter I shall mention only those features of recurrent importance in the pathological descriptions that follow.

THE NEURONES AND ITS CHANGES (Fig. 1)

The neurones vary in size, form and function, and all are exceedingly complex cells of whose working we are still largely ignorant. The work edited by Hydén (1967) reviews current knowledge of the neurones and traces the historical development of our understanding of this complicated and specialised cell. Investigation of the metabolism of neurones is clearly of great importance. We can look forward to the application of new techniques, e.g. those of histochemistry (Campa and Engel, 1970), which will elucidate the biochemical processes within the neurone

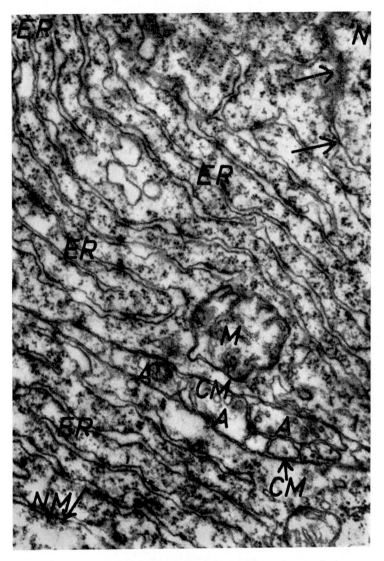

FIG. 1.—Electron microscope picture showing part of two large spinal neurones separated by cell membrane (CM). Between these two cells very fine axons pass (A). Note the laminated construction of the Nissl bodies separated here by a mitochondrion (M). E.R. = endoplasmatic reticulum, covered by ribosome granules which form the subunits of a Nissl body. N = nucleus, N.M. = nuclear membrane. The upper right arrows indicate the tortuous course of a nuclear membrane.

and which may show biochemical differences underlying differences in neuronal function.

Neurones have intense metabolic activity and are unusually susceptible to lack of glucose and oxygen, yet many must endure the life span of a human being, since, as far as we know, they are not formed after the neonatal period. When destroyed the cell body or perikaryon is not replaced and any injury is usually irreversible. When the axonic process is damaged the important change of central chromatolysis occurs in the cell body whilst the distal part of the axon undergoes the degeneration known as Wallerian degeneration. There are also changes in the central part of the axon, i.e. that part between the site of injury and the cell soma, but these changes are much less conspicuous (Cole, 1968).

Central Chromatolysis (Axonal Reaction) (Fig. 2)

This is the most important and distinctive variety of chromatolysis, a term which means the complete or partial loss of stainable Nissl substance from the cytoplasm of the cell body. In the spinal cord it is seen commonly in the motoneurones of the anterior horn and results from injury to the axon within the spinal cord, in the anterior spinal nerve root or in the peripheral nerve. It may also be seen in the large neurone cell bodies of the *nucleus dorsalis* (Clarke's column) when the appropriate axons of the posterior spinocerebellar tract are damaged, and in the smaller neurone cell bodies of the intermediolateral cell column when the preganglionic sympathetic nerve fibres are damaged either when traversing the white rami communicantes or elsewhere. The occurrence of central chromatolysis has provided a well-used method of tracing the origin of nerve tracts both in experimental animals and to a lesser extent in suitable human neuropathological material. The phenomenon itself has also attracted attention and the numerous light microscopical studies (Brodal, 1939; Cole, 1968; Cammermeyer, 1963) have now been supplemented by many ultrastructural observations (Torvik, 1972) and reports on the use of histochemical technique (Means and Barron, 1972). This body of experimental work must be used with caution in considering the cellular process of central chromatolysis in the human neurone. It must be emphasised that the phenomenon differs in detail according to the species, age of the animal, and the particular neurones concerned in the experiment. There is also a difference between those experiments which use crushing of a peripheral nerve trunk, when regrowth of the axon and recovery of the cell body is possible, and those experiments transecting the peripheral nerve trunk which usually leads to irreversible degeneration of the axon and cell body.

In the experimental animal central chromatolysis begins well within 12 hours, is well developed by the second day and has reached its maximum change in from 2–3 weeks. The most

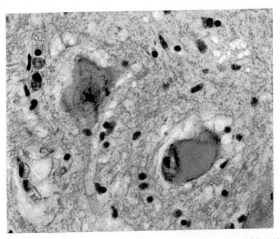

FIG. 2.—Anterior horn motoneurones in a case of peripheral neuritis. The cell body in the right lower quadrant shows central chromatolysis (axonal reaction). Note the disappearance of Nissl substance and eccentric position of the nucleus. Haematoxylin and eosin ×305.

obvious change is that the Nissl bodies disappear from the centre of the cell which swells and becomes more rounded whilst the nucleus is displaced away from the axon hillock to the margin of the cell and may change its shape, becoming oval. Cammermeyer (1963) has produced convincing evidence that some of these changes, notably the rounding of the cell and the displacement of the nucleus, are artefacts which can be avoided by meticulous control of tissue fixation. However the picture described above is that seen in human material and in most tissues of experimental animals.

The sequel to central chromatolysis in experimental animals is either the degeneration of the neurone or the gradual reversal

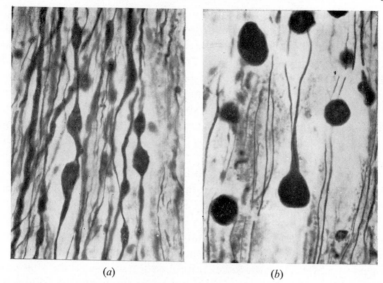

(a)   (b)

FIG. 3.—Longitudinal section of spinal cord showing nerve fibres stained by silver impregnation. Fig. 3a shows the early degenerative changes when the axons are swollen and beaded. In Fig. 3b the axons are severed with terminal swellings. Case of acute necrotic myelopathy. Holmes ×426.

of the changes over a period of up to 100 days. In human material, examined after periods of 4 months and 3 years, chromatolysis was present in the spinal motoneurones, but it was not seen in 4 cases with survival for 6, 8, 8 and 10 years (Hughes, 1966). These findings suggest that, in the human, central chromatolysis persists as a recognisable phenomenon for about 3 years after which the appearances in the motoneurone revert to normal.

Wallerian Degeneration

The most important degeneration effect seen in the white matter is that which occurs in the distal part of an axon following injury. Waller (1851) not only described these important changes but reported in an extensive series of publications how they could be used in tracing nerve-fibre tracts in the central nervous system. The fullest account of the use of this method is that of Cajal (1959) who had immense experience of degeneration and regeneration phenomena in the nervous system. The earliest changes are seen in the largest axons after approximately 24 hours. The axons first show beading (Fig. 3a), then in 4–8 days they break up into ovoid or spherical globules of axonic material (Fig. 3b). Further break-down occurs to a fine axonic dust which eventually disappears. During the degeneration of the nerve fibre the axonic material can be specially stained with silver by Nauta's method (Nauta and Ebbesson, 1970). This method and the developments of it have proved of great value in experimental neuroanatomy and also in human neuroanatomy when a short period of time has elapsed between the neurological destruction and death. In these circum-stances the Nauta technique is of more value than the older Marchi technique.

The nerve fibres ending within the central nervous system do so by forming unmyelinated terminations synapsing with another nerve cell body. Accompanying the other features of Wallerian degeneration, these terminations undergo swelling with drop-like fragmentation and bulbous changes of the *boutons terminaux*, which are the synaptic endings making contact with the cell body or its processes (Fig. 4). Silver impregnation enables these changes to be demonstrated and in this way nerve fibres can be followed to their terminations (Glees, 1946). This is possible within a few days of a lesion and before the Marchi technique shows degenera-tion of myelin. The modern development of this technique has been the use of the electron microscope to chart areas of neurones on which nerve fibres are terminating (Nauta and Ebbesson, 1970).

The myelin tube surrounding the axon undergoes dissolution at approximately the same rate. The first change of the myelin degeneration is seen as a "bubbly" state of the myelin tubes when examined by high power microscopy (Fig. 5). This is accompanied by irregular swelling of the myelin tubes which in transverse section may be twice their normal diameter. In longi-tudinal sections one can see that the swelling is uneven and takes the form of fusiform and balloon-like nodules. These nodules which mainly consist of breaking down myelin also enclose a small fragment of axonic material because the degenerating changes of the axon and the myelin proceed simultaneously. The myelin catabolism forms a series of chemical changes which have important histological accompaniments. The normal anisotro-pism of myelin, as seen with a polarising microscope, is lost. Neutral fat appears and the myelin breakdown products become sudanophilic. The Marchi method of staining degenerating myelin becomes positive about the tenth day and remains useful for a

year or even more (Smith, 1951). The method requires considerable skill and care; artefact staining is troublesome, but with
experience (Smith, 1956), does not limit the method. After three
or four weeks myelin breakdown is sufficiently advanced for tract
degeneration to be visible in the Weigert techniques in which the

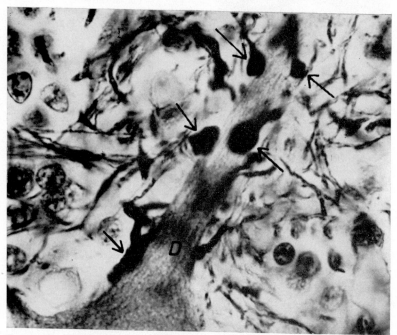

FIG. 4.—Dendritic portion of a spinal neurone covered with enlarged degenerating
synapses marked by arrows. The degeneration of synapses occurred after tri-cresyl-
phosphate poisoning. D = dendrite. To the left and right of the dendrite are neuroglial nuclei and branching axons. (Glees silver impregnation.)

preserved normal myelin is alone stained by the haematoxylin
method. The breakdown products of myelin are gradually
engulfed by histiocytes which are chiefly derived from the microglia (Fig. 6). Their complete removal is a process that lasts several
years, the final result being a slightly shrunken glial scar of astrocytes and their proliferated processes (Figs. 7 and 8).

THE GLIA AND ITS REACTIONS

The term *neuroglia* was bestowed by Virchow in 1846 (Virchow,
1862) *"eine Art von Kitt (Neuroglia) in welche die nervösen Ele-
mente eingesenkt sind"* (a sort of cement in which the nervous

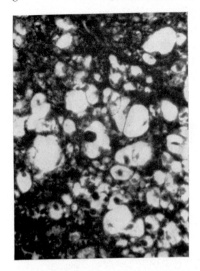

FIG. 5.—Photomicrograph from transverse section of spinal cord showing breaking down of myelin tubes, some of which are distended or have disappeared, leaving a round space which may contain a swollen axon. Case of acute necrotic myelopathy. Weil ×268.

elements are embedded). From the description that followed it is clear that Virchow also recognised actual glial cells but until the development of silver and gold impregnation techniques by Cajal and later by del Rio-Hortega the neuroglia could not be profitably studied.

Only when good electron micrographs became available almost half a century later was it appreciated that most of the background

FIG. 6.—Rosette of lipid phagocytes surrounding a small vessel and occupying a perivascular space in the spinal cord. This is a common phenomenon in the transport of lipid breakdown products. Haematoxylin and Van Gieson ×263.

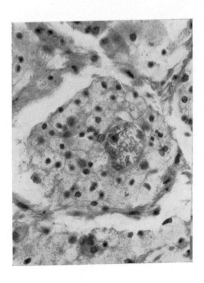

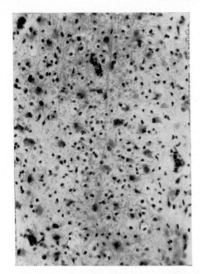

FIG. 7.—Photomicrograph from transverse section of spinal cord showing reactive astrocytes in the posterior columns. Many of the astrocytes are of the gemistocytic type and some have two nuclei. Luxol blue ×169.

material in the central nervous tissue consists of cell processes. By then three types of neuroglial cell had been separated, the astrocyte, the oligodendrocyte and the microglial cell.

FIG. 8.—Transverse section of spinal cord above a complete cord transection. The picture shows the end stage of astrocytic reaction when, after several years, the posterior columns have been transformed into an astroglial scar. The posterior columns are outlined by a mossy pattern of astrocytic fibrous gliosis. Haematoxylin and Van Gieson ×49.

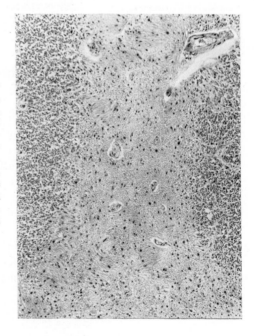

The Astrocyte

The main characteristics of the astrocyte were discovered by Cajal in the early part of this century. Cajal's gold-sublimate method stained the long radiating glial processes of the cells revealing their star-like form from which the name astrocyte is derived.

Two types of astrocyte may be identified in the spinal cord, the protoplasmic type found in the grey matter and the fibrous type found both in the white matter and in the grey matter. Numerous fine highly refractile fibres run through the cytoplasm of the cell body and the many branching processes of the fibrous astrocyte. There are few fibres in the processes of the protoplasmic astrocyte and the processes of this cell branch more often and at nearly a right angle so that the numerous branching fibres give a mossy background to the cell body. Both types have one thick process ending on a capillary wall as an expanded footplate. These end feet are so numerous on a capillary as to form a thick surrounding layer separating the vessel from the other components of the spinal cord. Electron microscopy has significantly increased our knowledge of the structure of the astrocyte (Peters *et al.*, 1970). With the electron microscope, the astrocyte appears large and pale with an irregular cell outline opening into many processes. Fibrils are numerous in the cell body and pass into the cell processes.

Despite much investigation, the function of both types of astrocyte can only be conjectured but in studying histological preparations of the spinal cord their reaction to injury or disease is constantly observed. The short account which follows deals with the changes that are most useful in diagnostic histology. It is thought that the reactive changes of both types of astrocyte are similar.

Gemistocytic astrocyte (*gemästet*, G. fattened) is a term disliked by purists but in general use. The cell is swollen, particularly the cytoplasm which has a hyaline appearance and eosin affinity. The nucleus moves to one side of the cell, and may enlarge and divide. This type of astrocyte (Fig. 7) is seen in a variety of cord disorders; it betrays a reaction to some process but has no known specific significance. The astrocyte undergoing this change does not appear irreversibly damaged and conceivably may return to its normal structure.

Clasmatodendrosis is a term introduced by Ramón y Cajal for a more severe reaction of the astrocyte which is generally regarded as irreversible. The cell body swells considerably and the processes are fragmented, leaving only irregular stumps and a dust of fibre fragments. The nucleus becomes small, dark and irregular. At a later stage the cell ruptures and both nucleus and cytoplasm disappear.

Fibrous gliosis is the final result of an astroglial reaction that falls short of irreversible damage to the cell. The reacting astrocyte enlarges and new fibres form whilst the original fibres elongate. A good deal of branching of fibres leads to a dense glial felt-work (Fig. 8). If this is of a random pattern it is called anisomorphous gliosis. Rather rarely in the spinal cord the fibres are orientated all in one direction, this arrangement being called isomorphous gliosis. If the cells themselves are so orientated they are called piloid astrocytes.

The Oligodendrocyte

Oligodendroglia were first clearly distinguished by Hortega (1921) who gave this name to the cells because of the paucity of their processes when stained by his metallic impregnation techniques. The oligodendrocyte has an analogous ensheathing function for the central axon to that which the Schwann cell has for the peripheral axon. Oligodendrocytes are prominent in the white matter of the spinal cord but are also seen in the grey matter in relation to axons and around neurone cell bodies as perineuronal satellites. By light microscopy the oligodendrocyte appears as a small cell with a round dark nucleus within a cell body which is polygonal or rounded with scanty cytoplasm and a few irregular processes. By electron microscopy (Peters *et al.*, 1970) the whole cell appears electron-dense and stands out from the paler astrocytes. The nucleus is round and dark with nuclear chromatin which tends to clump. The scanty cytoplasm is usually seen as a thin rim around the nucleus. It is dark mainly because of the abundance of rough-surfaced endoplasmic reticulum with many cisternae studded by ribosomes but also because of the electron density of the background cytoplasmic matrix. The Golgi apparatus is well developed. There are few cytoplasmic fibres and glycogen granules and mitochondria are not conspicuous. The formation and maintenance of the myelin sheath by the interfascicular oligodendrocytes is now well established and presumably this is the main function of oligodendroglia related to axons. The perineuronal satellite oligodendroglia are thought to have a role in the nutrition of the neurone cell body but as yet there is little positive evidence for this.

Changes in oligodendrocytes in diseases of the central nervous system are not obvious. They disappear when a severe lesion destroys grey or white matter and they are absent from the plaques of multiple sclerosis. In the condition progressive multi-focal leucoencephalopathy (Davies et al., 1973), in which myelin destruction is prominent, the nuclei of the oligodendrocytes are conspicuously occupied by virus particles.

Satellitosis is the name given to an increase in oligodendrocytes around a neurone cell body. In the author's experience this observation is of doubtful significance because of the difficulty in distinguishing perineuronal oligodendrocytes from other cells (e.g. lymphocytes or microglia) the nuclei of which may be similar to those of oligodendroglia.

The Microglia

Hortega in the years 1919–21 distinguished (del Rio-Hortega, 1932) the microglia cell from the phagocytic cells carried into the central nervous system in the blood stream or arising from vascular endothelial cells. It is thought that microglia are of mesodermal origin and invade the brain and spinal cord soon after birth. Their function in the normal state is obscure and they may be awaiting the stimulus of damage to undergo their striking and varied changes. The resting cell is of varying size and shape, a common form being an elongated cell with a fusiform nucleus, with very little cytoplasm and no obvious processes visible in general tissue stains. These resting forms are usually perivascular in distribution and are inconspicuous. Following trauma or disease and pre-eminently in acute infarction, the microglia proliferate rapidly, as is evidenced by the presence of numerous mitotic figures. Within three to four days the cells take up lipid, becoming rounded and foamy in paraffin-embedded material. These cells are termed lipid phagocytes or compound granular corpuscles and frequently these swollen phagocytes cluster around blood vessels in the form of a rosette (Fig. 6). Whether they discharge their load of lipid into the lumen of the vessel or whether the phagocytes themselves migrate into the blood stream with their burden is not known. This account of the normal state and of the potential activity of the microglial cell is probably that accepted by the majority of neuropathologists. There is however a substantial minority opinion that the bulk and perhaps all of the lipid phagocytes are derived from cells migrating into the central nervous system in response to tissue damage. The extreme view would deny the existence of microglia in normal central nervous tissues. The main current argument for this view is the difficulty by electron microscopy in separating a distinctive microglial cell. The accounts of Luse (1968) and of Peters *et al.* (1970) review the conflicting evidence of light and electron microscopy concerning the reality of microglia.

The Ependyma

The ependyma lines the central canal of the spinal cord but in the adult this is frequently closed or discontinuous. In embryological development the ependymal cells are ciliated but in the mature nervous system they are columnar cells with large oval basal nuclei. For a detailed account of ependyma and for a description of the ultrastructure of the ependymal cells, the reader is referred to Tennyson and Pappas (1968). There is also a valuable review by Fleischhauer (1972). Beneath the ependyma is a zone of glia intermediate between astrocytes and ependymal cells, and from this so-called subependymal glia, tumours occasionally arise and have histological characteristics reminiscent of their origin.

Corpora Amylacea

These large rounded hyaline bodies are named because they are stained by iodine, but they are not related to amyloid and do not contain fat. They are almost invariably associated with chronic degenerations of the spinal cord, whether due to a specific chronic disease or to the simple atrophy of old age. They frequently appear in a degenerating white matter tract and are very common as a peripheral rim to a senile spinal cord. Their presence and position is sometimes helpful in the diagnosis of chronic degenerative conditions of the spinal cord by providing another indication of the distribution of the degeneration. For a review of the histochemical and chemical nature of corpora amylacea the reader is referred to the account by Austin and Sakai (1972). From ultrastructural studies (Ramsey, 1965) it appears that corpora amylacea are formed as intracytoplasmic inclusion bodies within astrocytes.

Rosenthal Fibres

These strange structures are large carrot-shaped homogenous masses which stain strongly with eosin and with phosphotungstic-acid haematoxylin. In the spinal cord they are frequently seen in the walls of syringomyelic cavities and also within benign astrocytic tumours. Electron microscopy has shown that Rosenthal fibres are formed within the processes of astrocytes in which intense proliferation of glial filaments can be seen.

Arachnoid Plaques

When first encountered, arachnoid plaques (Fig. 9) surprise the novice neuropathologist. They are also encountered at laminectomy operations by puzzled junior neurosurgeons who excise them and send the material for histological section. These plaques consist of fatty deposits of usually structureless material in the arachnoid mater (Knoblich and Olsen,

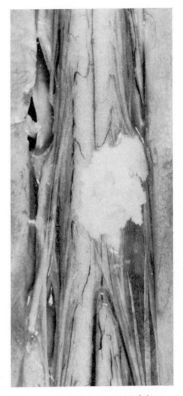

FIG. 9.—Anterior aspect of lower thoracic part of spinal cord showing a large arachnoid plaque.

1966). They are common in the elderly and may be very numerous. As far as is known they have no pathological significance.

REFERENCES

AUSTIN, J. H. and SAKAI, M. (1972). Corpora amylacea. In *Pathology of the Nervous System*, Vol. III, Chap. 212. Ed. by J. Minckler. New York: McGraw-Hill.

BLACKWOOD, W. and CORSELLIS, J. A. N. (1976). (Eds.) *Greenfield's Neuropathology*, 3rd edit. London: Edward Arnold.

BOURNE, G. H. (1968–72). (Ed.) *The Structure and Function of Nervous Tissue*, Vols. 1–6. New York: Academic Press.

BRODAL, A. (1939). Experimentelle Untersuchungen über retrograde

Zellveränderungen in der unteren Olive nach Läsionen des Klein-hirns. *Z. ges. Neurol. Psychiat.*, **166**, 646–704.

CAJAL, S. RAMÓN (1952). *Histologie du système nerveux de l'homme et des vertébrés*, Vols. 1 and 2. Madrid: Instituto Ramón y Cajal.

CAJAL, S. RAMÓN (1959). *Degeneration and Regeneration of the Nervous System*, Vols. 1 and 2. New York: Hafner.

CAMMERMEYER, J. (1963). Differential response of two neuron types to facial nerve transection in young and old rabbits. *J. Neuropath. exp. Neurol.*, **22**, 594–616.

CAMPA, J. F. and ENGEL, W. K. (1970). Histochemistry of motor neurons and interneurons in the cat lumbar spinal cord. *Neurology (Minneap.)*, **20**, 559–568.

COLE, M. (1968). Retrograde degeneration of axon and soma in the nervous system. In *The Structure and Function of Nervous Tissue*, Vol. 1, Chap. 7. Ed. by G. H. Bourne. New York: Academic Press.

DAVIES, J. A., HUGHES, J. T. and OPPENHEIMER, D. R. (1973). Richardson's disease (Progressive multifocal leukoencephalopathy). *Quart. J. Med.*, **42**, 481–501.

DEL RIO-HORTEGA, P. (1921). La glía de escasas radiaciones (oligo-dendroglía). *Bol. Soc. esp. Hist. nat.*, **21**, 63–92.

DEL RIO-HORTEGA, P. (1932). In *Cytology and Cellular Pathology of the Nervous System*, Vol. 2, p. 485. Ed. by W. Penfield. New York: Hoeber.

FLEISCHHAUER, K. (1972). Ependyma and subependymal layer. In *The Structure and Function of Nervous Tissue*, Vol. VI, Chap. 1. Ed. by G. H. Bourne. New York: Academic Press.

GLEES, P. (1946). Terminal degeneration within the central nervous system as studied by a new silver method. *J. Neuropath. exp. Neurol.*, **5**, 54–59.

GLEES, P. (1961). *Experimental Neurology*. Oxford: Clarendon Press.

HUGHES, J. T. (1966). Pathological findings following the intrathecal injection of ethyl alcohol in man. *Int. J. Paraplegia*, **4**, 167–175.

HYDÉN, H. (1967). *The Neuron*. Amsterdam: Elsevier.

KNOBLICH, R. and OLSEN, B. S. (1966). Calcified and ossified plaques of the spinal arachnoid membranes. *J. Neurosurg.*, **25**, 275–279.

LUBARSCH, O., HENKE, F. and RÖSSLE, R. (1955–58). In *Handbuch der Speziellen Pathologischen Anatomie und Histologie*, Vol. XIII. Ed. by W. Scholz. Berlin-Göttingen-Heidelberg: Springer.

LUSE, S. (1968). Microglia. In *Pathology of the Nervous System*, Vol. I, Chap. 44. Ed. by J. Minckler. New York: McGraw-Hill.

MEANS, E. D. and BARRON, K. D. (1972). Histochemical and histoiogical studies of axon reaction in feline motoneurones. *J. Neuropath. exp. Neurol.*, **31**, 221–246.

MINCKLER, J. (1968–72). (Ed.) *Pathology of the Nervous System*. Vols. 1–3. New York: McGraw-Hill.

NAUTA, W. J. and EBBESSON, O. E. (1970). *Contemporary Research Methods in Neuroanatomy*. (Proceedings of an International Conference at the Institute of Perinatal Physiology at San Juan in 1969.) Berlin: Springer.

PENFIELD, W. (1932). (Ed.) *Cytology and Cellular Pathology of the Nervous System*. Vols. 1–3. New York: Hoeber.

PETERS, A., PALAY, S. L. and WEBSTER, H. DE F. (1970). *The Fine Structure of the Nervous System*. New York: Hoeber.

RAMSEY, H. J. (1965). Ultrastructure of corpora amylacea. *J. Neuropath. exp. Neurol.*, **24**, 25–39.

SMITH, M. C. (1951). The use of Marchi staining in the later stage of human tract degeneration. *J. Neurol. Neurosurg. Psychiat.*, **14**, 222–225.

SMITH, M. C. (1956). The recognition and prevention of artefacts of the Marchi method. *J. Neurol. Neurosurg. Psychiat.*, **19**, 74–83.

TENNYSON, V. M. and PAPPAS, G. D. (1968). Ependyma. In *Pathology of the Nervous System*, Vol. 1, Chap. 43. Ed. by J. Minckler. New York: McGraw-Hill.

TORVIK, A. (1972). Phagocytosis of nerve cells during retrograde degeneration. *J. Neuropath. exp. Neurol.*, **31**, 132–146.

VIRCHOW, R. (1862). *Gesammelte Abhandlungen*, p. 890. Berlin: Max Hirsch.

WALLER, A. V. (1851). Nouvelle méthode pour l'étude du système nerveux applicable à l'investigation de la distribution anatomique des cordons nerveux. *C.R. Acad. Sci. (Paris)*, **33**, 606–611.

CHAPTER II

DEVELOPMENTAL AND CONGENITAL DISORDERS OF THE SPINAL CORD

The familial neuronal system degenerations peculiar to the spinal cord have so little in common with the various developmental and congenital disorders of the spinal cord that they are described in a separate chapter (Chapter III). Here we shall deal only with the developmental structural disorders of the spinal cord—a group of spinal cord abnormalities mainly manifest at birth.

We must first consider the normal development of the spinal cord and bear in mind that the structure of the adult cord is only exactly attained after a period of years and that the pace of development continuously declines. Consequently it is in the crowded events of intra-uterine life that we must seek the cause of the grosser developmental disorders. Readers wishing to amplify this short account of the embryology of the spinal cord should consult Keibel and Mall (1910–12), Keith (1948), Starck (1955), Blechschmidt (1961), and Langman (1968).

THE NORMAL DEVELOPMENT OF THE SPINAL CORD

The earliest primordial structure of the nervous system is the *neural plate*, a band of proliferated ectodermal cells arising in the midline of the embryonic disc. The folding of the two *neural folds* forms the neural groove and when the folds fuse the groove becomes the *neural tube*. From this neural tube the whole central nervous system develops, the differentiation of the caudal portion into the spinal cord being much less complex than the development of the brain. The *neural crest* arises by separation of cells from the dorsolateral aspect of the neural tube; these neural crest cells occupy the angle between the neural tube, the surface ectoderm and the body somites. From the neural crest develop the spinal ganglia whose central processes invade the spinal cord whilst their peripheral processes form the sensory nerves.

Development of Ependyma, Neurones and Neuroglia (Figs. 10, 11. 12 and 13)

When the neural tube is first formed, its wall is a single layer of columnar type cells, these cells being the inner layer of the infolded neural groove. These columnar cells multiply by mitotic division and presently three layers can be defined. Hiss (1889) and later Hardesty (1904) have interpreted these layers as follows, The innermost layer, which may be termed the *ependymal zone*, consists of a high columnar epithelium amongst which are other large round cells called by Hiss *"germinal cells"* and believed to give rise, by division and differentiation, to neuroblasts. Spongioblasts were thought to arise from the columnar cells of the ependymal zone and to differentiate into glial cells. The middle of the three layers, which may be termed the *mantle zone*, consists of densely packed layers of nuclei of cells destined to form both neurones and glia. These cells were thought to be derived partly from the cells of the ependymal zone and partly by self-replication. The third and outermost layer, which may be termed the *marginal zone*, has few nuclei but many processes from the cells of the mantle zone. This is the classical description (Clark, 1971) of early development of the central nervous system. In the spinal cord the ependymal zone ultimately becomes the central canal, the mantle zone gives rise to the neurones and glia whilst the marginal zone develops into the spinal-cord white matter.

Some details of the origin of the various cells and their disposition in the three zones have been modified (Langman, 1968) following the use of several modern experimental techniques. Colchicine and vincristine, which halt mitoses in the metaphase, when applied to early chick embryos cause a conspicuous appearance of arrested metaphase mitotic figures all within the ependymal zone. However, the measurement of nuclear DNA by microspectrophotometry demonstrates an increase in the DNA content of nuclei in the deeper mantle layer. The DNA in a nucleus increases during the interphase and prophase of mitosis finally

---

FIG. 10 (*see opposite*).—Section of spinal cord of chick after seven days of incubation. ×14 000. Note the elongated neuroblasts with their nuclei (N). L = lysosomes, M = mitochondria, MV = multivesicular body, G = Golgi apparatus, ER = endocellular reticulum. Left lower inset, magnified from framed portion of larger picture, shows the developing synapses. ×39 000. POST = post-synaptic membrane, SV = synaptic vesicles. Note the large Golgi apparatus in contrast to the small amount of the ER and the abundance of free ribosomes.

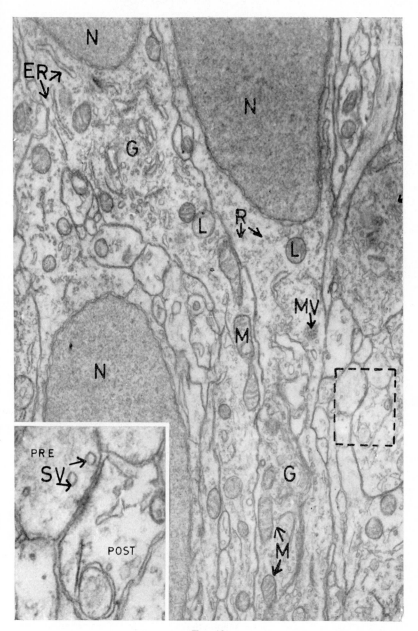

FIG. 10

reaching an amount which is twice the normal. This evidence suggests that the prophase of mitosis is seen in nuclei situated in the mantle zone. The problem has been further examined using tritiated thymidine, which labels radioactively the cells preparing for division at the time the thymidine is given. Thymidine, being an essential precursor of DNA, is incorporated into the newly synthesised DNA molecule. Using radio-autography, these cells and their descendants can be identified. By this method it has been shown that nuclei in the mantle zone take up DNA and then migrate to the ependymal zone where the metaphase of mitosis

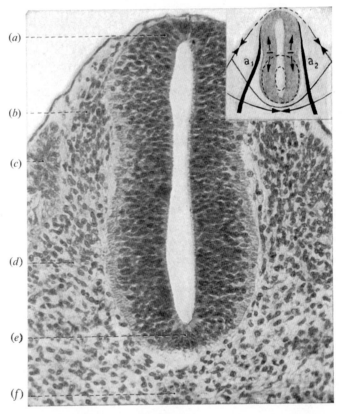

Fig. 11.—Early embryonic dorsum anlage of a *ca.* 3·7-mm. human embryo. The arrows in the small inset diagram indicate the moulding by differential growth that takes place in the neural tube. (*a*) Roof plate of neural tube; (*b*) neural crest sub-divided into neurotomes; (*c*) dorsal dermatomyotome edge of a somite; (*d*) meta-meric mesoderm; (*e*) floor plate, infrequent mitoses; (*f*) notochord.

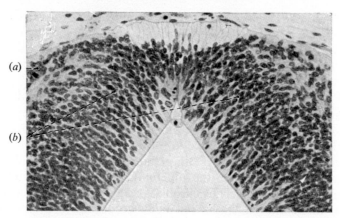

FIG. 12.—Dorsal zone of appositional growth of spinal cord in a 14-mm. human embryo. (*a*) Tissue sloughed off the neural tube laterally; (*b*) growth area with numerous mitoses.

takes place after which they return to the mantle zone. Electron microscopy has shown that at the stage of closure of the neural tube probably only one population of cells, which we should term *neuroepithelial cells*, is concerned. These are long cells forming a stratified epithelium and connected to each other at their inner

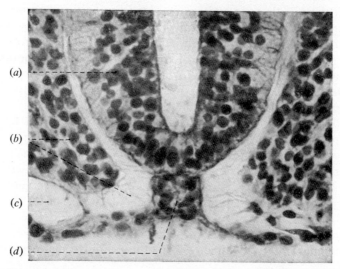

FIG. 13.—Appearance of grey and white matter in a human embryo with 13–14 pairs of somites. (*a*) Ventral horn; (*b*) zone of a sclerotome, *above* many nuclei, *below* fewer nuclei; (*c*) aorta still as a capillary; (*d*) notochord.

(luminal) ends by prominent terminal bars. After DNA synthesis the nucleus moves towards the lumen into the ependymal zone where the metaphase of mitosis takes place (resembling the "germinal cell" of Hiss) following which the nucleus returns into the mantle zone.

When the neural tube is formed and in the chick embryo at about the second day there is a differentiation of some of the neuroepithelial cells into neuroblasts recognisable initially by a single short process directed towards the lumen of the neural tube. From tritiated thymidine studies, it is thought that no replication occurs after the differentiation of a neuroepithelial cell into a neuroblast. The neuroblast then develops into a neurone with differentiation of the cell body according to the neuronal type, and with growth of the axon first into the enlarged marginal zone and finally to its remote destination. As a consequence of the continuous production of neuroblasts there is considerable moulding of the neural tube which grows extensively in its lateral aspects but scarcely at all dorsally and ventrally. Consequently the tube in cross section is first a narrow slit, then becomes diamond-shaped and finally fuses throughout nearly all of its extent to form the posterior median septum, the only part remaining open being the central canal. The spinal cord neurones develop from the mantle zone and are moulded by their growth into the anterior, posterior, and lateral grey columns. The white matter of the cord gradually enlarges by growth of fibres from the neurones of the grey matter of the spinal cord, of the posterior spinal ganglia, and of those growing caudally from the brain. The white matter develops in the position formerly occupied by the marginal layer of the neural tube.

The neuroglia is considered to arise from primitive cells known as spongioblasts but the recognition of these early glial forms is difficult and consequently the early development of glia is still poorly understood. It is thought that both the types of astrocyte and the oligodendrocyte arise from the primitive spongioblast. The microglia are first seen in the spinal cord beneath the pia and around blood vessels, and are thought to be derived from mesoderm and to migrate into the central nervous tissues. The ependyma is derived directly from the primitive neuroepithelial cells.

The origin of the meninges of the spinal cord is still in some dispute. The dura probably arises from mesoderm but there is good evidence that the leptomeninges arise from the neural crest. The neural crest is formed from the most laterally situated part of the neural tube and these cells migrate laterally and ventrally to form the posterior root ganglia and the ganglia of the autonomic nervous system. They also probably give rise to the leptomeninges, because if the neural crest is excised from an experimental animal not only do the posterior root ganglia and the autonomic ganglia fail to develop but the outgrowing fibres from the anterior nerve roots are not clothed by Schwann cells.

Nomenclature

It may be helpful first to define some of the terms commonly used in describing developmental and inherited disorders affecting the spinal cord.

The word *congenital* is useful when taken to mean "present at birth" but it is unwise to attribute a more extensive meaning to the term. A developmental defect, presenting at birth as a congenital lesion, may be caused by an exogenous agent acting in intrauterine life. Conversely the group of inherited neuronal system degenerations described in Chapter III are due to some inborn error of development (or of maintenance) of the nervous system but these diseases may not be apparent at birth.

To avoid similar inconsistencies, the word *acquired* should be used only to mean that the defect appeared after birth.

The word *genetic* (synonymous in my usage with "inherited" and "familial") is useful to describe conditions in which an abnormality of a gene can be reasonably postulated. Park (1964), who discusses the semantics of these terms, suggests the use of the term *non-genetic* when a developmental disorder can be ascribed to a known etiological agent. Unfortunately only a few such agents (rubella virus, thalidomide) have been recognised as causes of spinal and developmental disorders. We can only speculate about the large remainder of conditions which have to be classified according to the anatomical structure of the abnormality.

Rubella Embryopathy

In 1941 Gregg, an ophthalmologist in Australia, published a paper showing the connection between congenital cataract and congenital heart disease and the occurrence of German measles in the mother during the first two months of her pregnancy.

Following up this astute observation, from 1942 to 1946 Swan (1949) carried out a survey of the incidence of maternal rubella and congenital malformations in South Australia. There were congenital malformations associated with maternal rubella in 101 cases and of these spina bifida occulta was present in three cases, spastic diplegia in one case and hemiparesis in one case. A further report of spina bifida was made by Krause (1945). The importance of these early observations has been amply substantiated. The situation is that if the mother develops rubella before the end of the second month of her pregnancy there is a 5 per cent risk of fetal abnormality and a 10 per cent risk of the child being stillborn. The mechanism is thought to be the infection of the embryo by the rubella virus which, being of a benign nature, acts in this way rather than causing the death of the embryo. For a congenital disorder to appear there must be a disturbance of development at this early phase. Many abnormalities may be present, the commonest being cataracts, eye deformities, and congenital heart disease. In the nervous system, in addition to those mentioned, mental deficiency is common and there may be retinal changes.

Apart from rubella only the cytomegalovirus has been shown in man to cause developmental abnormalities affecting the nervous system. Intrauterine infection with the cytomegalovirus may cause microcephaly, hydrocephaly, porencephaly and periventricular calcification. No particular spinal cord developmental disorder seems to have been attributed to this virus. Evidence incriminating other viruses is unconvincing. Elizan et al. (1969) made a careful comparison between a series of 54 mothers who had given birth to children with neural malformations and a series of normal controls. Examination of paired maternal sera using 16 viral antigens failed to demonstrate any clear association of the neural malformation with maternal viral infection during pregnancy.

Thalidomide-induced Deformities

In November 1961 a paper read at Düsseldorf by Dr. W. Lenz reported the occurrence of malformed children born to women who had taken the hypnotic drug thalidomide in the early stages of pregnancy. Thalidomide, alpha N-phthalimido glutarimide, was sold in West Germany as "Contergan", in Great Britain as "Distaval", and in U.S.A. as "Kevadon". Originally developed by Grunethal in 1958 it had in Germany within twelve months achieved a very wide sale as a safe reliable hypnotic. It was freely available without prescription to the general public but also was very popular with practitioners and was widely used in general hospitals and in mental institutions. In this way the stage was set for the appearance of a new disease, which in the years 1959, 1960 and 1961 startled and perplexed German paediatricians by the appearance of the rare abnormality phocomelia in epidemic form. Shortly after the communication of Lenz came reports of cases in Australia (McBride, 1961) and in Great Britain (Speirs, 1962). A few cases have occurred in Sweden, Belgium, Switzerland, U.S.A. and Canada (Taussig, 1962). It was estimated by Lenz (1962) that in West Germany since 1959 between two and three thousand thalidomide-deformed babies have been born. The drug was withdrawn from distribution in Germany on 25 November 1961 and from Great Britain on 2 December 1961. The number of cases which occurred in Great Britain was probably of the order of one thousand and in a survey conducted by the Ministry of Health (1964) 894 cases of significant deformity were reviewed.

Clinical features.—Wiedemann (1961), in reporting the first large series of 33 abnormal children, described accurately the malformations encountered. Although a wide spectrum of developmental faults were seen the most striking feature was the type of limb deformity. The common form was phocomelia, in which a more or less rudimentary hand arose directly from the distal end of a shoulder bone without intervening elbow and wrist joints. Similar deformity was sometimes present in the legs but less frequently and less severely. In the most severe cases the state of amelia was present. The external ears were often deformed or absent and a facial haemangioma was situated on the forehead, nose and upper lip.

Pathological findings.—Few detailed autopsies have so far been reported and in many accounts the main concern has been in the external abnormalities and those of the viscera. Through the courtesy of Professor W. Krücke I was able to examine the spinal cords of several cases gathered at the Max-Planck Institute for Nervous Diseases in Frankfurt. In these dissected and serially sectioned specimens the brachial plexus was often present despite a rudimentary limb. The nerve fibres in the brachial plexus were diminished and in the cervical enlargement the anterior horn was of a simpler configuration than is normal.

The results of several experimental observations are now available and Somers (1962) has produced in rabbits limb deformities identical with those in human cases. The circumstantial evidence is overwhelming that thalidomide acts on the developing embryo to produce multiple abnormalities, the most characteristic being phocomelia.

Myelodysplasia (Spinal Dysraphism)

Myelodysplasia, myeloschisis, and spinal dysraphism are names given to a group of disorders in which the neural groove fails to develop normally into the spinal cord and other posterior midline structures.

Von Recklinghausen (1886) pointed out that if the normal formation of the neural tube by folding of the neural plate was arrested then an incomplete neural tube with a posterior deficiency of structures would result. He suggested that arrested development of the neural tube could account for the various types of myelodysplasia. Among others, Sternberg (1929), from work on young human embryos, confirmed the views of Von Recklinghausen. This explanation of the etiology of the myelodysplasias still appears without discussion in many standard textbooks (Potter, 1961; Willis, 1962; Morison, 1970; Potter and Craig, 1976).

Much earlier Morgagni (1769) had suggested that the pressure of the fluid from a case of hydrocephalus could distend the spinal canal into a similar watery malformation. This suggestion of Morgagni was forgotten when subsequently the embryological development of the neural tube was studied. However Gardner in a long series of papers (best reviewed in Gardner, 1973) has put forward a theory of maldevelopment of the neural tube that recalls the early conjectures of Morgagni. He considers that most of the developmental disorders under discussion arise by the distension of a neural tube which formed without any posterior deficiency. The views of Gardner and the many reports quoted by him (Gardner, 1973) deserve to be studied in detail. Varying degrees of distention or rupture of the neural tube would explain meningocele, meningomyelocele and myelocystocele. Elaborations of this pathogenic mechanism are made by Gardner to explain hydromyelia, syringomyelia, iniencephalus, diastematomyelia, and the Klippel-Feil syndrome. Whilst it is likely that there are links between some of these conditions it remains to be shown that all of them are caused by overdistension with or without rupture of the primitive neural tube. Meanwhile it seems best to review the various structural malformations under the familial morphological headings. Where there is evidence of etiology this will be indicated. The following references are suggested for further reading: Ingraham *et al.* (1943), Cameron (1957*a*, 1957*b*), Smith (1965), James and Lassman (1972), Emery and Lendon (1973).

Spina Bifida

This is the name given to incomplete closure of the vertebral canal which commonly is seen as posterior spina bifida in which there is a defect of the vertebral laminae. This defect may occur at any level of the spinal column but is most common in the lumbosacral region. The laminar defect may be the only serious abnormality and such cases, recognised by X-rays, are called *spina bifida occulta*. The incidence of this condition is difficult to estimate and some clinical surveys of radiography have given an incidence as high as 10 per cent. In spina bifida occulta the overlying skin may show tell-tale blemishes such as hair, a dimple or a port-wine naevus. There may be fibrous adhesions between the spinal cord and the subcutaneous tissues. The spinal cord itself may be affected, with gliosis and cavitation. These cases are those which have clinical neurological impairment, the most common feature being difficulty of sphincter control. When spina bifida is associated with a posterior cystic lesion the condition is called *spina bifida cystica*. All these cases present with a bulging sac in communication with the open spinal canal. The customary nomenclature derives from the contents of this sac and the terms meningocele, meningomyelocele, and meningomyelocystocele are commonly used. In series of cases in which the contents of the sac have been carefully examined meningocele has been shown to be rare. Usually some part of the spinal cord can be found within the sac.

Anterior spina bifida is the condition in which the vertebral bodies are malformed and the spinal canal has an anterior deficiency. These cases may have fistulous connections between the spinal canal and either the mediastinum or intestine. There may be entodermic cysts within the spinal canal. These cases, which present as space-occupying lesions, will be described in Chapter X.

Meningocele

This name is given to cases in which spina bifida is associated with a bulging subcutaneous sac the main contents of which are meninges and fluid. The incidence of this type of spinal dysplasia is not known but it is rare in cases (possibly the most severe) in which the sac has been carefully examined histologically. The leptomeninges lining the sac give a smooth glistening internal surface. The skin covering the sac may be normal or more usually is thin and atrophic without appendages. Excoriation is frequent and creates a serious hazard of infection. Histologically the

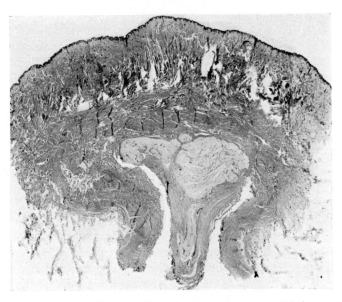

FIG. 14.—Section of surgically excised meningomyelocele sac. This is a common finding, when a portion of gliotic central nervous system suggestive of spinal cord but containing no surviving neurones, is present within the sac. These cases merge imperceptibly into the category of meningomyelocystocele. Haematoxylin and Van Gieson × 5.

meningeal layers can usually be recognised but the dura often blends with fibrous tissue in the dermis. It is not uncommon to find structures such as nerve roots and there is no exact boundary from the next group to be considered.

Meningomyelocele (Fig. 14)

In a case with this degree of deformity there is, within the sac, a lump of central nervous tissue (the plaque) which histologically represents a damaged spinal cord with nerve roots. Frequently the whole spinal cord is a mass of fibrous gliosis with no evidence of intact neurones. Often there is partial preservation of cord structure and the ependymal-lined central canal can frequently be recognised. These cases merge into the more severe abnormality of myelocystocele. The neurological deficit varies according to the anatomical defect. Skin cover in this type is poorer than in the meningoceles and secondary infection is common.

Meningomyelocystocele

This is always a serious developmental disorder because the meningeal sac contains a badly malformed spinal cord. Usually only the anterior half of the cord has a roughly normal anatomy. The posterior part is absent or spreads out to merge with the inner

TABLE (From Emery and Lendon, 1973)

Type and incidence of major cord lesion in 100 cases

Numbers of cases showing major cord lesions

with form of cord	in region		
	cranial to plaque	plaque region	caudal to plaque
Normal	14	1	15
Hydromyelia	29	0	0
Syringomyelia	14	2	0
Winged cord	6	3	0
Absent canal	0	1	0
Multiple canals	0	1	15
Dorso-ventrally elongated canal	0	13	0
Open plate—symmetrical	0	30	0
asymmetrical	0	5	0
Hemimyelocele	0	9	0
Double cords	31	22	25
Double canal	5	5	27
Unclassifiable	1	8	18
All forms	100	100	100

wall of the sac. The central nervous tissue is mainly glia but ependyma can usually be seen often as a dilated central canal widely open posteriorly. In all these cases the neurological deficit and prognosis are grave. Hydrocephalus and the Arnold–Chiari deformity are very commonly associated, adding further problems in management.

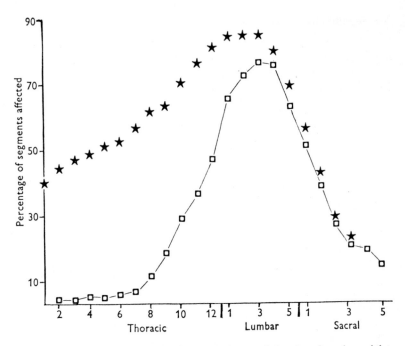

Graph to show extent of overt plaque (□) and gross deformity of cord cranial to plaque (★). Percentile distributions from 100 cases.
(From Emery and Lendon, 1973)

The pathology of the contents of the sac in these three conditions has been recently reported by Emery and Lendon (1973) who describe their findings in 100 necropsies of meningomyelocele, a term they use for all "open cystic or non-cystic lesions associated with spina bifida". Thus they would use "meningomyelocele" to include cases of meningocele and meningomyelocystocele. This report of Emery and Lendon (1973) merits careful study since previously only Marsh *et al.* (1885) and Leveuf *et al.* (1937) had investigated large series of cases.

In Emery and Lendon's series there were 43 female and 57 male children. The interesting feature of their findings is the widespread nature of the spinal cord abnormality, not only in the exposed part of the cord (the plaque region) but above and below. Their Table on page 29 shows the types of abnormality found, and their graph on page 30 the extent and the situation of the overt plaque and the accompanying gross deformity of the cord found cephalad to the plaque. Diplomyelia was found in 31 per cent of the cases and syringomyelia in 14 per cent. The complicated pathological findings in these cases suggest multiple linked factors in the causation of the malformations rather than a single causal mechanism.

Diplomyelia and Diastematomyelia (Figs. 15 and 16)

These terms are used synonymously for a disorder in which some part of the spinal cord is divided longitudinally into two

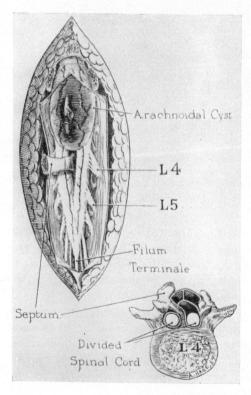

FIG. 15.—Drawings of operative findings in a case of diastematomyelia. A bony and fibrous septum splits the cord below an arachnoid cyst. Note the abnormally low location of the conus medullaris in the spinal canal. The smaller picture shows a cross-section view of the pathological findings.

similar structures. This interesting anomaly has attracted considerable interest and among others there are full accounts by
Weil and Matthews (1935), Herren and Edwards (1940), and
Perret (1960). The incidence of the condition in spina bifida
cystica has been dealt with above.

Spina bifida is commonly present. The spinal canal is abnormal
varying from being abnormally wide to being duplicated. When

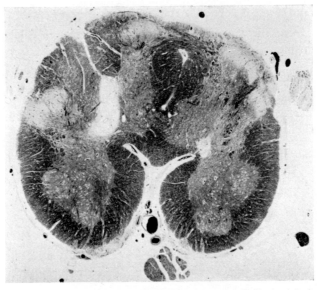

FIG. 16.—Transverse section, stained for myelin, through the spinal cord of a case of
diastematomyelia. The picture shows the situation in the lumbosacral enlargement
where the two halves of the partially divided cord are united by their incomplete
medial portions. Weil ×7.

there are two canals these are separated by an antero-posterior
septum made of fibrous tissue, cartilage or bone. The meninges
are usually duplicated, the pia always, the arachnoid and dura in
about half the cases. The duplication of the spinal cord occurs
throughout about ten spinal segments usually below the mid-
thoracic region. In a case examined by the author, hydromyelia
(dilatation of the central canal) was present in the upper thoracic
region. As one proceeded caudally, there came a point where the
dilated and elliptical canal divided into two (Fig. 16). Further
still there were two almost complete cords joined posteriorly and

each rotated through 90°. As often happens the medial anterior horns and roots of each cord were underdeveloped. Many of these cases are seen in childhood with a varying degree of neurological deficit. Some attain adult life, a few with no apparent disability.

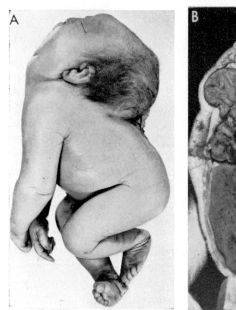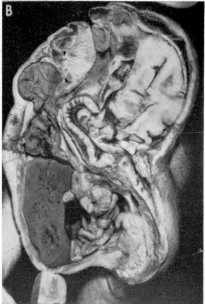

FIG. 17.—Iniencephalus due to confluence of cranial and spinal cavities. A, exterior view; B, sagittal section showing relation of cavity of skull to spinal canal. The brain is cut slightly to the right of the midline. Cerebellum, pons, medulla, and spinal cord are absent. All abdominal viscera except the liver are within the thoracic cavity because of an associated defect of the diaphragm.

Iniencephalus and the Klippel–Feil Syndrome

Iniencephalus is thought (Gilmour, 1941) to be the most extreme form of the disorder described by Klippel and Feil (1912). The name iniencephalus derives from the deformity of the neck (*inion*) (Fig. 17) but in this gross malformation there is also abnormality of the brain, spinal cord, viscera and locomotor system. The neck is short and, due to marked retroflexion, the face looks upwards. The spinal canal is grossly malformed and, due to absence or fusion, there are fewer vertebrae. The spinal cord is always maldeveloped and may be absent.

In the Klippel–Feil syndrome there is shortness and webbing of the neck due to maldevelopment of the cervical vertebrae. The bodies of these may be fused and posterior spina bifida is usually present. Because of the abnormal spinal canal there are frequently neurological signs referable to the cervical cord.

Syringomyelia

This disorder is usually distinguished from hydromyelia (dilatation of the central canal) and from longitudinal cysts caused by tumours, vascular softenings and injuries. So defined we have a primary spinal cord disease whose pathological basis is the development of progressive spinal cord cavitation in the form of a syrinx. The condition was first described by Portal (1803) and the name was suggested by Ollivier (1824). The disease was studied exhaustively by Schlesinger (1895) whose monograph is an excellent account. The subject was reviewed by Ostertag (1956). The reports of Netsky (1953) and of Feigin *et al.* (1971) described the clinical features and necropsy findings in eight and sixteen cases.

Clinical course.—The disease first becomes clinically manifest in the second or third decade though often a feature such as scoliosis has been present earlier. The usual course is slow but with relentless progression of neurological deficit appropriate to the central cavitation. Males and females are equally affected.

Pathological findings (Fig. 18).—Macroscopically the distended spinal cord is fluctuant but collapses on cutting. A perfect central

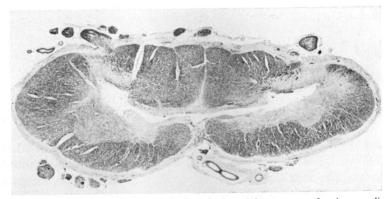

FIG. 18.—Transverse section through the spinal cord from a case of syringomyelia. The syrinx is here (in the cervical cord) symmetrical, involving both posterior horns and the grey commissure. The syrinx has collapsed *post-mortem.* Weil × 6.

cavity is rather rare; the usual appearance is a slit passing trans-versely through the cord and being often quite asymmetrical. The cavity wall may have a whitish or faintly yellowish appearance. The fresh cyst fluid is usually clear and may be similar in com-position to cerebrospinal fluid. It may be yellow and rarely (Perot *et al.*, 1966) haemorrhage may occur into the syrinx, a complication originally described by Gowers (1904). The extent of the syrinx is extremely variable but usually at least half the cord is involved. An extension into the medulla (syringobulbia) is common and sometimes there are two or more separate cavities in the spinal cord and brain stem.

Histologically the extent of the syrinx can be more clearly appreciated. The grey commissure is regularly destroyed but in the asymmetrical extensions one or both of either anterior or posterior horns may be affected. The position and extent of the white matter destruction is also variable. A common site is the white matter near a posterior root entry where the slit may reach the pia mater. The cavity wall consists of a glial layer of variable thickness and is often mixed with connective tissue. This may be only a few collagenous strands around blood vessels but sometimes there is a thick lining of vascular connective tissue. Ependyma as an inner lining is only present where the syrinx wall approaches the central canal. In this situation a part of the syrinx takes ependyma as its internal layer, but elsewhere the syrinx and the central canal may be quite distinct. A feature of the syrinx wall are small abnormal (peripheral type) nerve bundles probably arising from the nearby nerve roots and ramifying in the connective tissue (Hughes and Brownell, 1963).

Theories of etiology.—Secondary syringomyelia and hydro-myelia will be discussed later. The main problem is the patho-logical mechanism of "primary" syringomyelia. These cases, provided they are carefully distinguished from hydromyelia, are not associated with developmental abnormalities. Feigin, Ogata and Budzilovich (1971) found no association in 16 cases and this has been my experience. The nature of the syrinx fluid suggests strongly a communication with the cerebrospinal fluid. Possibly there are several alternative sites for this communication. Gardner (1973) believes that a communication exists between the fourth ventricle in the medulla and the syrinx in the spinal cord. However in many cases histological sections of the intervening tissue have failed at necropsy to demonstrate this connection.

Given a communication between syrinx and ventricle or sub-arachnoid space one must explain why the syrinx fills and enlarges. Pressure waves have been suggested either from arterial pulsation (e.g. from choroid plexus) or from an increase in venous pressure within the spinal canal and cranium, due to human activities (e.g. coughing, straining, etc.) which normally cause a displacement of cerebrospinal fluid upwards through the foramen magnum. The recurrence of such pressure changes would explain the enlargement of the syrinx in syringomyelia.

Secondary Syringomyelia

This term should be used for longitudinal cysts secondary to clearly evident causes. Tumours, trauma, adhesive arachnoiditis, haematomyelia and vascular softenings account for most cases and in many cases the cyst is small and scarcely justifies the name of syringomyelia. However in intrinsic cord tumours the associated cystic lesion may be extensive and progressive; in these cases the cyst contains a high-protein fluid secreted in some way by the intrinsic tumour.

Poser (1956) has reviewed the association between syringomyelia and neoplasms. Out of 254 cases of syringomyelia with autopsy reviewed by him 40 (16.4 per cent) had an associated intramedullary tumour while out of 209 cases of intramedullary tumours there was an incidence of 31 per cent of syringomyelia. Syringomyelia can be caused by extrinsic tumours as in the case of Kosary et al. (1969) who found an occipital meningioma. The syringomyelia found after traumatic paraplegia will be described in Chapter V.

Syringomyelia has been occasionally described following adhesive arachnoiditis (Schwarz, 1898; Nelson, 1943) and a recent case with necropsy was reported by Appleby et al. (1969). In this case, which followed tuberculous meningitis, the authors considered that there was a communication to the syrinx from the fourth ventricle via a patent central canal.

Carroll (1967) described syringomyelia following an attack of acute anterior poliomyelitis and reviewed other case reports of this association.

Hydromyelia

The term hydromyelia should be reserved for dilatation of the central canal of the spinal cord. It is a common condition which in a minor degree, particularly in the upper cervical region, can be found in otherwise normal spinal cords from persons living normal life span without evidence of neurological disease. However hydromyelia is very common in association with spina bifida occulta, spina bifida cystica (meningomyelocele), the Arnold–Chiari syndrome, and diastematomyelia. Thus there is an important correlation between hydromyelia and developmental malformations of the neural tube, a correlation which is absent in syringomyelia (primary and secondary) as defined above.

Developmental Abnormalities of the Neurenteric Canal

The neurenteric canal, in the presomite stage of a vertebrate embryo, is a short-lasting communication between the yolk sac and the caudal end of the neural groove. Its remnants should be sought (Bremer, 1952) near the tip of the coccyx and in this location would open any fistula arising from a normally sited neurenteric canal. In practice midline fistulae at other levels may occur and these may be persistent ectopic or accessory neurenteric canals. Keen and Coplin (1906) described a fistula which, arising from the rectum, passed through a malformed sacrum and between the roots of the cauda equina to end at the skin in a piloid opening. In a case of Saunders (1943) a similar tract was associated with anterior and posterior spina bifida and with diastematomyelia. The two halves of the spinal cord were separated by the persistent neurenteric canal. Bremer (1952) considers this arrangement to be usual in diastematomyelia and the median spur seen in this condition to be formed from the neurenteric canal.

Further cases with reduplication of the gut and enteric cysts both with connection to the spinal meninges through anterior spina bifida have been described by McLetchie et al. (1954), Rhaney and Barclay (1959), Silvernail and Brown (1972) and Millis and Holmes (1973). More common than neurenteric fistulae are cysts whose entodermic lining suggests a similar origin. They may be small and commonly are seen in the filum terminale and cauda equina. Occasionally they are large and they may occur in other locations as in the large thoracic cyst described by Holcomb and Matson (1954).

REFERENCES

APPLEBY, A., BRADLEY, W. G., FOSTER, J. B., HANKINSON, J. and HUDG-SON, P. (1969). Syringomyelia due to chronic arachnoiditis at the foramen magnum. *J. neurol. Sci.*, **8**, 451–464.

BLECHSCHMIDT, E. (1961). *The Stages of Human Development before Birth.* Basel: Karger.

BREMER, J. L. (1952). Dorsal intestinal fistula; accessory neurenteric canal; diastematomyelia. *Arch. Path.*, **54**, 132–138.

CAMERON, A. H. (1957a). The Arnold-Chiari and other neuro-anatomical malformations associated with spina bifida. *J. Path. Bact.*, **73**, 195–211.

CAMERON, A. H. (1957b). Malformations of the neuro-spinal axis, urogenital tract and foregut in spina bifida attributable to disturbances of the blastopore. *J. Path. Bact.*, **73**, 213–221.

CARROLL, J. D. (1967). Syringomyelia as a possible complication of poliomyelitis. *Neurology (Minneap.)*, **17**, 213–215.

CLARK, W. E. LE G. (1971). *The Tissues of the Body*, 6th edit. Oxford: Clarendon Press.

ELIZAN, T. S., AJERO-FROEHLICH, L., FABIYI, A., LEY, A. and SEVER, J. L. (1969). Viral infection in pregnancy and congenital CNS malformations in man. *Arch. Neurol.*, **20**, 115–119.

EMERY, J. L. and LENDON, R. G. (1973). The local cord lesion in neurospinal dysraphism (meningomyelocele). *J. Path.*, **110**, 83–96.

FEIGIN, I., OGATA, J. and BUDZILOVICH, G. (1971). Syringomyelia. The role of edema in its pathogenesis. *J. Neuropath. exp. Neurol.*, **30**, 216–232.

GARDNER, W. J. (1973). *The Dysraphic States*. Amsterdam: Excerpta Medica.

GILMOUR, J. R. (1941). Essential identity of Klippel-Feil syndrome and iniencephaly. *J. Path. Bact.*, **53**, 117–131.

GOWERS, W. R. (1904). Syringal haemorrhage into the spinal cord. Lecture VIII in *Lectures on Diseases of the Nervous System*. Second series. London: Churchill.

HARDESTY, J. (1904). On the development and nature of the neuroglia. *Amer. J. Anat.*, **3**, 229–268.

HERREN, R. Y. and EDWARDS, J. E. (1940). Diplomyelia (duplication of the spinal cord). *Arch. Path.*, **30**, 1203–1214.

HISS, W. (1889). Die Neuroblasten und deren Entstehund im embryonalen Mark. *Arch. Anat. Entwicklungsgesch.*. 249–300.

HOLCOMB, G. W. and MATSON, D. D. (1954). Thoracic neurenteric cyst. *Surgery*, **35**, 115–121.

HUGHES, J. T. and BROWNELL, B. (1963). Aberrant nerve fibres within the spinal cord. *J. Neurol. Neurosurg. Psychiat.*, **26**, 528–534.

INGRAHAM, F. D., SWAN, H., HAMLIN, H., LOWREY, J. J., MATSON, D. D. and SCOTT, H. W., Jr. (1943). *Spina Bifida and Crania Bifida.* Cambridge, Mass: Harvard University Press.

JAMES, C. C. and LASSMAN, L. P. (1972). *Spinal Dysraphism. An account of 100 cases of spina bifida occulta submitted to laminectomy.* London: Butterworth.

KEEN, W. W. and COPLIN, W. M. L. (1906). Sacrococcygeal tumour (teratoma). *Surg. Gynec. Obstet.*, **3**, 662–671.

KEIBEL, F. and MALL, F. P. (1910–12). *Manual of Human Embryology.* Philadelphia: Lippincott.

KEITH, A. (1948). *Human Embryology and Morphology*, 6th edit. London: Edward Arnold.

KLIPPEL, M. and FEIL, A. (1912). Un cas d'absence des vertèbres cervicales avec cage thoracique remontant jusqu'à la base du crâne. *Nouv. Iconogr. Salpêt.*, **25**, 223–250.

KOSARY, I. Z., BRAHAM, J., SHAKED, I. and TADMOR, R. (1969). Cervical syringomyelia associated with occipital meningioma. *Neurology (Minneap.)*, **19**, 1127–1130.

KRAUSE, A. C. (1945). Congenital cataracts following rubella in pregnancy. *Ann. Surg.*, **122**, 1049–1055.

LANGMAN, J. (1968). Histogenesis of the central nervous system. In *The Structure and Function of Nervous Tissue*, Vol. 1, Chap. 2. Ed. by G. H. Bourne. New York: Academic Press.

LENZ, W. (1962). Thalidomide and congenital anomalies. *Lancet*, **1**, 45.

LEVEUF, J., BERTRAND, I. and STEINBERG, H. (1937). *Études sur le spina bifida.* Paris: Masson.

MCBRIDE, W. G. (1961). Thalidomide and congenital abnormalities. *Lancet*, **2**, 1358.

MCLETCHIE, N. G. B., PURVES, J. K. and SAUNDERS, R. L. DE C. H. (1954). The genesis of gastric and certain intestinal diverticula and enterogenous cysts. *Surg. Gynec. Obstet.*, **99**, 135–141.

MARSH, H., GOULD, A. P., CLUTTON, H. H. and PARKER, R. W. (1885). Report of a committee nominated to investigate spina bifida and its treatment by the injection of Dr. Morton's codo-glycerine solution. *Trans. clin. Soc. Lond.*, **18**, 339–418.

MILLIS, R. R. and HOLMES, A. E. (1973). Enterogenous cyst of the spinal cord with associated intestinal reduplication, vertebral anomalies, and a dorsal dermal sinus. *J. Neurosurg.*, **38**, 73–77.

MINISTRY OF HEALTH (1964). Reports on public health and medical subjects. N. 112. *Deformities Caused by Thalidomide.* London: H.M.S.O.

MORGAGNI, G. B. (1769). *The Seats and Causes of Diseases Investigated by Anatomy*, Vol. 3. Translated by Benjamin Alexander. London: A. Millar and T. Cadell.

MORISON, J. E. (1970). *Foetal and Neonatal Pathology*, 3rd edit. London: Butterworths.

NELSON, J. (1943). Intramedullary cavitation resulting from adhesive spinal arachnoiditis. *Arch. Neurol. Psychiat.* (*Chic.*), **50**, 1–7.

NETSKY, M. G. (1953). Syringomyelia. *Arch. Neurol. Psychiat.* (*Chic.*), **70**, 741–777.

OLLIVIER, C. P. (1824). *De la moelle épinière et ces maladies.* Paris: Crevot.

OSTERTAG, B. (1956). Die Einzelformen der Verbildungen (einschliesslich Syringomyelie). In *Handbuch der Speziellen Pathologischen Anatomie und Histologie*, Vol. XIII/4, pp. 363–601. Ed. by W. Scholz. Berlin-Göttingen-Heidelberg: Springer.

PARK, W. W. (1964). The classification of developmental defects. *Lancet*, **2**, 579–580.

PEROT, P., FEINDEL, W. and LLOYD-SMITH, D. (1966). Hematomyelia as a complication of syringomyelia. Gowers syringal haemorrhage. *J. Neurosurg.*, **25**, 447–451.

PERRET, G. (1960). Symptoms and diagnosis of diastematomyelia. *Neurology* (*Minneap.*), **10**, 51–60.

PORTAL, A. (1803). *Cours d'anatomie médicale*, 5t. Paris: Baudouin.

POSER, C. M. (1956). The relationship between syringomyelia and neoplasms. Springfield, Illinois: Thomas.

POTTER, E. L. (1961). *Pathology of the Fetus and Infant*, 2nd edit. Chicago: Year Book Medical Publishers.

POTTER, E. L. and CRAIG, J. M. (1976). *Pathology of the Fetus and the Infant*, 3rd edit. Chicago: Year Book Medical Publishers.

RHANEY, R. and BARCLAY, G. P. T. (1959). Enterogenous cysts and congenital diverticula of the alimentary canal with abnormalities of the vertebral column and spinal cord. *J. Path. Bact.*, **77**, 457–471.

SAUNDERS, R. L. DE C. H. (1943). Combined anterior and posterior spina bifida in living neonatal human female. *Anat. Rec.*, **87**, 255–278.

SCHLESINGER, H. (1895). *Die Syringomyelie.* Leipzig: Franz Deuticke.

SCHWARZ, E. (1898). Ein Fall von Meningomyelitis syphilitica mit Höhlenbildung im Rückenmark. *Z. klin. Medi.*, **34**, 469–525.

SILVERNAIL, W. I. and BROWN, R. B. (1972). Intramedullary enterogenous cyst. *J. Neurosurg.*, **36**, 235–238.

SMITH, E. D. (1965). *Spina Bifida and the Total Care of Spinal Myelomeningocele.* Springfield, Ill.: Thomas.

SOMERS, G. F. (1962). Thalidomide and congenital abnormalities. *Lancet*, **1**, 912–913.

SPEIRS, A. L. (1962). Thalidomide and congenital abnormalities. *Lancet*, **1**, 303–305.

STARCK, D. (1955). *Embryologie.* Stuttgart: Thieme.

STERNBERG, H. (1929). Über Spaltbildungen des Medullarrohres bei jungen menschlichen Embryonen, ein Beitrag zur Entstehung der Anencephalie und der Rachischis. *Virchows Arch. path. Anat.*, **272**, 325–374.

SWAN, C. (1949). Rubella in pregnancy as an aetiological factor in congenital malformation, stillbirth, miscarriage and abortion. *J. Obstet. Gynaec. Brit. Emp.*, **56**, 341–363, 591–605.

TAUSSIG, H. B. (1962). A study of the German outbreak of phocomelia. *J. Amer. med. Ass.*, **180**, 1106–1114.

VON RECKLINGHAUSEN, F. (1886). Ueber die Art und die Entstehung der spina bifida, ihre Beziehung zur Rückenmarks—und Darmspalte. *Virchows Arch. path. Anat.*, **105**, 296–330.

WEIL, A. and MATTHEWS, W. B. (1935). Duplication of the spinal cord, with spina bifida and syringomyelia. *Arch. Path.*, **20**, 882–890.

WIEDEMANN, H. R. (1961). Himweis auf eine derzeitige Häufung hypo- und aplastischer Fehlbildungen der Gliedmassen. *Med. Welt (Stuttg.)*, **37**, 1863–1866.

WILLIS, R. A. (1962). *The Borderland of Embryology and Pathology*, 2nd edit. London: Butterworth.

CHAPTER III

NEURONAL SYSTEM DEGENERATIONS

The nervous system is strangely affected in a group of diseases which can be termed "neuronal system degenerations". The characteristic of these diseases is a selective degeneration of certain anatomical patterns of neurones in the central or peripheral nervous system. In this chapter the diseases of this type which involve the spinal cord are described. The majority of these conditions are familial inherited diseases although there is one conspicuous example (motor neurone disease) which commonly occurs without a familial background.

We shall describe the following diseases: Friedreich's ataxia (hereditary spinocerebellar ataxia), Strümpell's familial spastic paraplegia (hereditary spastic paraplegia), Werdnig–Hoffmann disease (hereditary spinal muscular atrophy), hereditary motor neurone disease, motor neurone disease (Charcot–Marie–Tooth disease, (peroneal muscular atrophy).

Before these conditions are described some comment on the etiological possibilities of the whole group is appropriate. The inheritance of these conditions suggests that a genetically deter-mined metabolic defect may underlie the neuronal degeneration. Inherited metabolic defects are well known in certain childhood cerebral diseases and Crome and Stern (1972) list 200 examples and give brief accounts of the specific biochemical error if this is known. To date very few of these discovered biochemical abnor-malities have caused a syndrome involving the spinal cord. There are however two examples of considerable interest, one due to deficiency of β-lipoprotein (Bassen–Kornzweig syndrome) and another associated with an abnormality of glycine metabolism. In Leigh's disease (Leigh, 1951) in which carbohydrate metabolism is abnormal the exact metabolic disorder is not yet known.

The interesting diseases of kuru and Jakob–Creutzfeldt disease now have claims to be considered among infectious diseases and will be described in Chapter VI.

Friedreich's Ataxia (Hereditary Spinocerebellar Ataxia)

Of the various types of hereditary spinocerebellar degeneration this form is the commonest, the best documented, and was the earliest recognised. When Friedreich of Heidelberg described the clinical and pathological features of this disease in a series of papers in 1861, 1863, and 1876, he was separating the disease by its hereditary background from locomotor ataxia, which at that time included most of the ataxias diagnosed. The first report in England was that of Gowers (1880) and in America that of Smith (1885). For a review of the genetic, clinical, and pathological aspects of the disease the reader is referred to Greenfield (1954). Very full pathological descriptions were made by Mott (1907), Spiller (1910), Lambrior (1911) and Estable (1931–32).

Genetics and clinical course.—The evidence suggests that Friedreich's ataxia may be transmitted either by a simple autosomal recessive gene or by an autosomal dominant gene, the instances of the former being about twice that of the latter mode of inheritance. Consanguinity of the parents is much commoner than in the population as a whole and instances of the disease in twins have several times been reported. The onset of the disease is usually before the age of 20; it was found by Bell and Carmichael (1939) that the mean age of onset in 320 cases of the recessive type was 11.75 years and in 84 cases of the dominant type was 21.4 years. These authors described the usual clinical course of steady progression and the average age of death in their first group was 26.5 years and in their second group 39.5 years.

The predominant clinical symptoms and signs are those of ataxia. This first appears as an ataxia of gait and then causes clumsiness of the hands and later dysarthria. Nystagmus is present and sometimes there are attacks of vertigo. The tendon jerks are lost at an early stage and sometimes the plantar responses are of extensor type. Deformity is common, *pes cavus* being the most often noted, but there is also claw-hand and kyphosis. Heart disease is associated and the common cause of death is heart failure.

Pathological findings.—The main findings are long-tract degenerations in the spinal cord (Fig. 19). These occur in the gracile and cuneate tracts of the posterior columns, the anterior and posterior spinocerebellar tracts and the lateral corticospinal tracts. The atrophy of the posterior spinocerebellar tract is greater than the anterior and is associated with depletion and loss of nerve cells

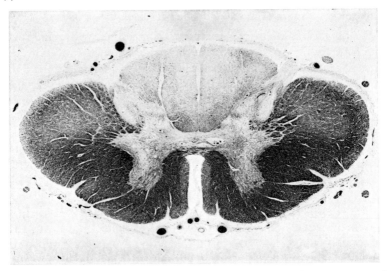

FIG. 19.—Friedreich's ataxia. Transverse section, stained for myelin, at T1 segmental level. There is degeneration of the posterior columns, of the corticospinal tracts and of the spinocerebellar tracts. Weil ×8.

in Clarke's column which shows gliosis. The posterior nerve roots are atrophied with nerve fibre loss and loss of nerve cells in the posterior root ganglia. In a study of the peripheral nervous system in 22 cases (Hughes *et al.*, 1968) a severe depletion of large myelinated fibres was found whilst the small-diameter unmyelinated nerve fibres were preserved. The detailed neuronal degeneration in the brain was also studied in the author's laboratory in 15 cases.

In the brain stem the degeneration of the sensory pathway continues with cell loss and gliosis of the gracile nuclei (severely affected) and the cuneate nuclei (moderately affected). Degeneration is seen in the medial fillet and is severe in the anterior region (gracile) but less conspicuous in the posterior (cuneate) region. The sensory roots of the trigeminal and glossopharyngeal nerves are degenerated as are the optic nerves (severely in half the cases) and both the vestibular and cochlear components of the auditory nerves. In the cerebellum the Purkinje cells, the granule cells, the stellate cells and the basket cells appear normal. However, the dentate nuclei show severe cell loss and gliosis and this is associated with marked degeneration of the superior and inferior cerebellar peduncles. The corticospinal tract degeneration could be seen in the pyramids of the medulla and occasionally in the pons but not in the cerebral peduncles of the midbrain. The giant pyramidal cells of the motor cortex were depleted.

Outside the nervous system the only constant finding has been a severe myocardial degeneration (Russell, 1946) with characteristics of a primary muscle degeneration.

Atypical Cases of Friedreich's Ataxia

The widespread changes described above from an experience of many necropsies of the disease indicates that some features thought to be rare are actually common in the disease. Optic atrophy, which was described (Andre-van Leeuwen, 1949) as a rare associated condition, is probably present in the late stage of most cases. In the families of Biemond (1928) and Spillane (1940) some of the affected members have Friedreich's ataxia and others peroneal atrophy. In the case of Hunt (1921) myoclonus was a feature of the disease and Roussy and Levy (1926) described a syndrome associated with Friedreich's ataxia in which some cases had amyotrophy.

Hereditary Spastic Paraplegia (Strümpell's Familial Spastic Paraplegia)

In 1880 Strümpell reported two brothers who developed a mild spastic paraparesis and in 1886 he reported the post-mortem findings in one of these cases and in 1904 the necropsy findings in a further case. Further accounts have been made by Schwarz (1952), Dick and Stevenson (1953), Schwarz and Liu (1956), and Behan and Maia (1974).

Genetics and clinical course.—In most of the families described, the inheritance can be explained by a simple dominant gene. Examples of recessive and sex-linked recessive inheritance have been reported but sometimes the diagnosis on these cases may not be correct.

The onset of the disease is in the second or third decade of life but occasionally earlier. The symptoms are of a slowly progressive weakness of the lower limbs which on examination shows an upper motor neurone paresis. The clinical course is quite benign and scarcely shortens life.

Pathological findings.—The spinal cord shows degeneration of the long tracts, the most constantly affected being the lateral corticospinal tracts below the medulla. Occasionally the tract degeneration can be demonstrated higher in the brain stem and Schwarz and Liu noted loss of Betz cells. Other tracts of the cord involved are the gracile and cuneate fasciculi of the posterior column and occasionally other long tracts. Developmental disorders of the cerebrum and cerebellum have also been found.

Werdnig–Hoffmann Disease (Hereditary Spinal Muscular Atrophy)

The literature on this subject begins in 1891 when Werdnig (1891) an obscure neurologist in Gratz described the clinical features of progressive weakness beginning in the lower limbs in two brothers, one of whom died at the age of 3 years. The autopsy demonstrated neuronal loss in the anterior horns associated with muscular atrophy and these features have since become pathognomonic of this condition. A further report was made by Werdnig in 1894 describing the clinical findings of six children, in two of whom complete necropsy studies were available. The eponymous use of Hoffmann's name dates from a series of papers beginning in 1893 (Hoffmann, 1893) reporting six cases in four different families in which the family histories revealed a total of 21 relatives suspected of the disease. These early papers contain an excellent account both of the clinical and pathological aspects of the condition which Werdnig called hereditary progressive muscle atrophy. Greenfield and Stern (1927) reported the postmortem findings of four cases of the disease together with a comprehensive review of the previous published necropsied cases. The most recent full review of the subject is that of Byers and Banker (1961) who described 52 cases with autopsy examinations in 18. The account that follows, whilst in accordance with the author's own experience, is largely taken from this latter paper. The subject was reviewed by Oppenheim in 1900 but this paper, based only on clinical findings without any pathological confirmation or an account of the subsequent clinical course, fails to establish Oppenheim's contention that there was a benign form of the disease. This confusion makes it undesirable to use the term Oppenheim's disease or Oppenheim's syndrome.

Clinical course.—The age of the patient at the onset of the disease ranges from intra-uterine life to the second year. This early onset is quite usual and inquiry often elicits the information that the quickening movements felt by the pregnant mother have become less apparent towards term. A few cases appear later and these tend to progress more slowly. There seems no obvious difference between the rapidly progressive cases and the slowly progressive cases and the separation of a benign group called Kugelberg–Welander disease seems unjustified (Munsat *et al.*, 1969). After birth the onset of the disease is seen as weakness first in the legs and then involving the arms, ending finally in a severe paresis of all four limbs and trunk. The diaphragm has always been reported as escaping the paralysis. The child adopts a characteristic posture with the arms abducted from the shoulder and flexed at the elbow joints. The legs are in a frog-like position with external rotation and abduction at the hip joint, with flexion at the hip joint and the knee joint. Fasciculation is seen in the muscles and there is loss of the tendon reflexes. The other reflexes are normal and there is no sensory loss or sphincter disturbance. There is no evidence of an upper motor neurone lesion such as hyper-reflexia or clonus. Tremor was described in the original cases of Werdnig and was a common feature in the series of Byers and Banker. This tremor, occurred throughout active movement and also during the maintenance of posture. It was a simple fine tremor persisting at the same rate and amplitude throughout movements and was thought by these workers to be due to muscle weakness. The electromyograph shows fasciculation of the muscles tested. Plain X-rays show poorly developed muscle shadows.

Genetic considerations.—Byers and Banker found, as had previous observers, that the inheritance was compatible with an autosomal recessive gene. Many of the cases were siblings, one pair were second cousins and the disease had occurred in an aunt and two great aunts. The corrected incidence of affected children as a proportion of healthy siblings was 32.1 per cent, and this was close to that theoretically calculated for an autosomal recessive gene.

Pathological findings. (i) *Cerebrum, cerebellum and brain stem.*— The pathological changes found in the cerebrum and cerebellum are astrocytic and microglial proliferation in the cortex, internal nuclei and dentate nucleus of the cerebellum. These changes are probably due to anoxia rather than to the specific disease process. No abnormality is seen in the Betz cells and, in the white matter, myelination appears normal. In the brain stem the only abnormalities found are in the cranial nerve motor nuclei. These changes are

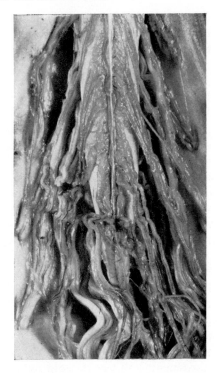

FIG. 20.—Anterior aspect of the spinal cord from a case of Werdnig-Hoffmann disease. Note the underdeveloped anterior spinal nerve roots which are thread-like in comparison with the posterior spinal nerve roots.

seen in the motor nuclei of the fifth, sixth and seventh nerves, nucleus ambiguus, supra-spinal nucleus, and twelfth nerve nucleus. The changes consist of central chromatolysis, nerve-cell depletion with gliosis, and neuronophagia.

(ii) *Spinal cord* (Fig. 20).—In all the cases the myelination of the spinal cord has been normal. The grey matter of the posterior horn, the lateral horn, and of Clarke's column are always normal. The abnormal findings are seen in the anterior horn cells at all levels of the spinal cord. The chief abnormality is the loss of the large motor neurones. Many of the cells are altered in shape being rounded with peripheral Nissl substance, and an eccentric nucleus. Some cells show ballooning as in severe central chromatolysis. Other anterior horn cells are pyknotic and shrunken and the variety of changes suggests a pattern of degeneration ending in pyknotic shrunken cells. At all segmental levels neuronophagia can be seen. Corresponding to these degenerative neuronal changes and presumably secondary are some reactive changes of astrocytes and microglia around the anterior horns. This fibrous gliosis is easily seen in Holzer stains. No abnormality is seen in either the posterior roots or their ganglia or in the sympathetic ganglia. The anterior roots are shrunken both within and outside the cord, and there is an increase of connective tissue corresponding to depletion of nerve fibres and an increase in Schwann cells. Sections of peripheral nerves show loss of myelinated fibres in the motor parts of the nerve with increase in Schwann cells and connective tissue fibrosis.

(iii) *Muscle.*—The appearances on section of muscles are well known in this disease, for many biopsies have been made to supplement the data from necropsies. The muscle fibres show atrophy in large connected groups, the distribution being suggestive of motor unit atrophy and reminiscent of motor neurone disease. These small fibres are usually rounded in shape and contain myofibrils and an increase of sarcolemmal nuclei. Between atrophied fasciculi are groups of normal muscle fibres, and these include some which are larger than normal, rounded in shape with centrally placed nuclei. It is important not to mistake these for the appearances of a myopathy. The muscle spindles are prominent with normal intrafusal fibres, but the small nerve endings in the muscle show loss of fibres. These atrophic changes are present in all muscles except the diaphragm and the strap muscles of the neck. The tongue is variably involved but sometimes no changes are present. The ultrastructure of the denervated muscle fibres (Hughes and Brownell, 1969) does not differ from the appearances in other causes of denervation.

Hereditary Motor Neurone Disease

The common sporadic form of motor neurone disease will be described later. Here will be mentioned the occurrence of combined lower motor neurone and upper motor neurone disease principally of the spinal cord but occurring in adults in a familial setting. In the majority of the world population these families of hereditary motor neurone disease are rare. Studies of their inheritance have usually pointed to the operation of an autosomal dominant gene with incomplete penetrance and varying expressivity. The situation is dramatically different in the Chamorro population of Guam and in Rota in the Mariana Islands. In this ethnic group, according to Kurland (1957), the incidence is 420 per 100,000 with a high preponderance of familial examples.

The disease in these familial cases appears to be identical with that occurring sporadically and the pathological reports are also remarkably similar.

Hereditary Combined Neurological System Degeneration

Under this term I propose to consider a variant of hereditary motor neurone disease first completely described by Hirano *et al.* (1967). The authors of this paper reported a new case and reviewed the pathological findings in other similar cases from three families. All the pathological features of motor neurone disease were present including pyramidal tract degeneration, absence of spinal motor neurones, wasting of anterior spinal nerve roots and denervation atrophy of the skeletal muscles. In addition all the cases had degeneration of the posterior white columns, and of both the anterior and posterior spino-cerebellar tracts. Clarke's column was severely degenerated. One of the interesting features of the condition was the presence in many of the surviving anterior horn motor neurones of hyaline intracytoplasmic material. In a study of a case of this disease (Hughes and Jerrome, 1971) this material was shown, by electron microscopy, to consist of bundles of neurofilaments approximately 10 nm in diameter and morphologically similar to normal neurofilaments.

Motor Neurone Disease

The current practice of including under this name progressive muscular atrophy, amyotrophic lateral sclerosis and progressive bulbar paralysis has convenience and emphasises the unity of the group, but many pathologists mourn the older nomenclature. Historically the three types were recognised as distinct diseases. Progressive muscular atrophy is associated with the names of Aran and Duchenne, amyotrophic lateral sclerosis was described by Charcot and Joffroy (1869), and the bulbar disease by Déjerine (1883). For a full review of the literature the reader is referred to Colmant (1958). A recent description of the pathological changes in the CNS is that of Brownell *et al.* (1970).

Clinical course.—The disease occurs in the third, fourth and fifth decades with a predominance in males. In the majority of cases there is no familial tendency but an identical disease has occasionally occurred with a strong family history.

The wide spectrum of clinical presentation and course arises from three fundamental clinical features:

1. Progressive lower motor neurone paralysis of the arms;
2. Progressive upper motor neurone paralysis of the legs;
3. Progressive lower motor neurone paralysis of the motor cranial nerves.

The most common combination of clinical signs are those of 1 and 2, and this combination was that originally described by Charcot and Joffroy. However, each of the three types may occur separately, and in every other combination. In the relatively pure types, the cases of upper motor neurone type (amyotrophic lateral sclerosis) progress more swiftly than the so-called progressive muscular atrophy.

Findings in the spinal cord.—Macroscopically the spinal cord appears generally rather atrophied but the pathognomonic appearance is the wasting of the anterior nerve roots which is particularly seen in the cervical enlargement. On cutting across the cord the grey outline of the degenerated corticospinal tracts can often be seen in the lateral columns.

Microscopically, the striking changes are the long-tract degeneration (Fig. 21), the loss of neurones from the anterior horns and the degeneration of the anterior spinal nerve roots. The long-tract degeneration, seen in Weigert preparations but also in Marchi, always affects the corticospinal tracts, both in the lateral white columns and in the uncrossed tracts of the anterior white columns. Although the corticospinal tracts are always well outlined by degeneration there is usually a lesser amount of degeneration in the spinocerebellar tracts. Other tracts may also degenerate, since the anterior and lateral columns are frequently pale throughout in contrast to the normal appearance of the anterior columns.

The changes in the grey matter, although greatest in the cervical enlargement, are seen at all segmental levels. The changes beyond dispute are the depletion of neurones from the anterior horn; the loss being most evident in the posterolateral cell column. The remaining neurones may be shrunken and the Nissl substance may be abnormal. Loss of neurones from the lateral and posterior horns is disputed and the cells of Clarke's column are usually normal. In these respects motor neurone disease differs from diseases such as poliomyelitis, syphilitic amyotrophy and cases of vascular diseases affecting the spinal cord. In all these conditions the region of damage is variable and may include all the grey matter and adjacent white matter. The additional difference in these disorders is that there is tissue destruction and following the removal of the damaged tissue the anterior horn and any other affected region becomes shrunken as a whole. In motor neurone disease the absent neurones are replaced by gliosis, but without shrinkage or deformity of the architecture of the grey column. The anterior spinal cord nerve roots are atrophied usually at all segmental levels. Both nerve fibres and myelin tubes are absent and the roots are

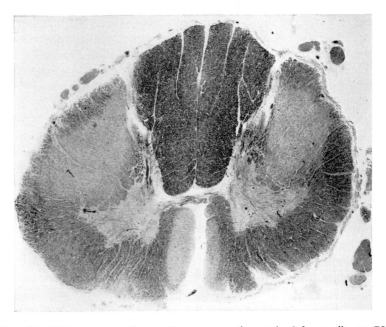

FIG. 21.—Motor neurone disease. Transverse section, stained for myelin, at C5 segmental level of a case of motor neurone disease. Note the preservation of the posterior columns. Although the majority of the fibres of the anterior and lateral columns appear affected the anterior and lateral cortico-spinal tracts are the worst affected and are distinctly outlined. Weil ×9.

shrunken with an increase in connective tissue. The posterior roots are normal.

Findings outside the spinal cord.—The white matter degeneration of the corticospinal tract can be traced backwards in medulla, pons, midbrain and even faintly in the internal capsule, but the intensity of the abnormality diminishes. The motor nuclei of the brain stem show similar changes to those in the spinal cord. The peripheral nerves show atrophy of their motor components and the muscles show characteristic denervation atrophy.

Etiology of motor neurone disease.—This remains completely unknown although naturally a wide variety of causes have been put forward. The theories are reviewed by Colmant (1958). Perhaps the most interesting feature is the link with inherited diseases afforded by rare examples of motor neurone disease with a definite genetically determined familial occurrence. A therapeutic trial of levodopa in ten patients (Mendell *et al.*, 1971) failed to give any improvement.

Charcot–Marie–Tooth Disease (Peroneal Muscular Atrophy)

This is a slowly familial disease characterised by muscle wasting affecting all four limbs but particularly the legs and particularly the peroneal group of muscles. It begins either in the first or second decade and is transmitted by an autosomal dominant gene or occasionally a recessive gene. The predominant features are motor weakness and wasting, to which are added sensory disturbance chiefly loss of joint and position sense.

Literature

The early reports of this disease are scattered throughout many nineteenth century medical journals and the literature is reviewed by Hughes and Brownell (1972) who added a report of the clinical and necropsy findings in four cases. Only 7 previous case reports with necropsy studies were found (Virchow, 1855; Friedreich, 1873; Marinesco, 1894; Sainton, 1899; Déjerine and Armand-Delille, 1903; Marinesco, 1928; Alajouanine *et al.*, 1967). The famous report of Charcot and Marie (1866) is of historical importance because their clinical description of five cases drew attention to the disease which in France is still called "Maladie de Charcot–Marie". In the same year Tooth (1886) published a very full account of the clinical findings in several cases whose study formed the basis of a Cambridge University thesis. These cases were later reported in a medical journal (Tooth, 1887).

Pathological Findings

The only relevant tract degeneration seen in the central nervous system can be explained as a secondary Wallerian degeneration from a disease process primarily affecting the posterior root ganglia and the peripheral nerves. Moderate fibre degeneration in the posterior columns is present in all cases and this affects the gracile more than the cuneate fasciculi. This degeneration corresponds in intensity to the degeneration found in the posterior roots. It is less than the degeneration seen in severe tabes dorsalis, in Friedreich's ataxia, and above a complete cord transection.

The other constant feature seen in the spinal cord is loss of motor neurone cell bodies from the anterior horns. This loss is less severe than that seen in motor neurone disease and has features such as central chromatolysis not seen in that disease, while neuronophagia (found regularly in motor neurone disease) is not observed. These differences from motor neurone disease may indicate a difference in the progression of the disease in an individual neurone. The disease may begin in the cell body in motor neurone disease, whereas in peroneal muscular atrophy the axon outside the central nervous system may be the first affected. Other differences may be attributable to the very chronic course of peroneal muscular atrophy. The very large numbers of corpora amylacea in the anterior horns indicate a degeneration with a long time course.

The histological examination of the peripheral nervous system is the most productive. The spinal nerve roots, both anterior and posterior, consistently show degeneration. This is less in the posterior roots than is seen in tabes dorsalis and in Friedreich's ataxia, and less in the anterior roots than is seen in motor neurone disease. This difference of severity may be due to the extreme chronicity of peroneal muscular atrophy. Death is usually due to some other incidental condition and the disease may not become fully manifest as do the other fatal neurological degenerations.

The posterior root ganglia always show extensive changes with loss of neurone cell bodies and degenerative changes in those remaining. The proliferation of the capsule cells surrounding the vacant space of a cell body is conspicuous and similar to that seen in Friedreich's ataxia. The peripheral nerves always show severe degeneration with fibrosis which seems out of proportion both to the clinical disability and to the secondary degeneration seen in the spinal cord and skeletal muscle. Why this disproportion exists requires explanation. Perhaps in this disease we see in the peripheral nerve trunk a summation of neurological degenerations. Here is combined all the afferent degeneration seen in Friedreich's ataxia and the efferent degeneration seen in motor neurone disease. We know that the afferent fibres make up the bulk of peripheral nerve trunks even of those nerves which are termed "motor". It seems likely that the degeneration of all these fibres results in the excessive fibrotic atrophy of the peripheral nerves seen in this condition. The degeneration of the peripheral nerves is worse than in Friedreich's ataxia (where the efferent motor fibres are intact) and very much worse than in motor neurone disease (where sensory afferent fibres are unaffected).

The changes in the skeletal muscle are constant except in their degree, which varies. Small groups of atrophied muscles suggest denervation and very characteristic is the extreme atrophy of muscle fibres in atrophic groups. Sometimes only sarcolemmal nuclei within a sarcolemmal membrane can be identified, giving a spurious impression of multinucleated giant cells. Inflammatory cells were very rarely seen and the muscle fibres never showed any changes of a myopathy or of a dystrophy. A constant finding (Hughes and Brownell, 1972) is atrophy of the muscle spindles, with thickening of the capsule and fibrous tissue proliferation within the capsule.

Abetalipoproteinaemia (Bassen–Kornzweig Syndrome)

Bassen and Kornzweig (1950) first described the association of malformed erythrocytes (acanthocytes) with retinitis pigmentosa and a progressive neuropathic ataxia, and ten years later Salt *et al.* (1960) showed that in a similar case the serum contained virtually no β-lipoprotein. Many cases have now been described (Crome and Stern, 1972) and a large literature of cases has accumulated. The inheritance is by an autosomal recessive gene and consanguinity in the parents is common.

The condition is diagnosed during life by the association of retinitis pigmentosa, acanthocytosis, steatorrhoea, ataxia and neuropathy. The serum lipid changes are characteristic. The serum cholesterol is below 70 mg/100 ml and the serum phosopholipids are low. Immune electrophoresis of serum shows the absence of β-lipoprotein. By ultracentrifugal analysis the serum levels of α-lipoprotein are shown to be low and chylomicrons and pre-β-lipids are absent.

The pathology of the disease was studied by necropsy in a 36-year-old woman by Sobrevilla *et al.* (1964). Heart, ovarian and renal lesions were present. In the spinal cord there was degeneration of the posterior columns and the spinocerebellar tracts and neurone loss from the anterior grey horns and the cerebellar cortex. The peripheral nerves were also degenerated.

Hyperglycinaemia

Many families of cases having hyperglycinaemia have been reported and the disorder can be subdivided into a ketotic and a non-ketotic form (Crome and Stern, 1972). In the ketotic form there is severe mental retardation with other features such as osteoporosis, thrombocytopenia and neutropenia. These associated features are absent in the non-ketotic form who exhibit lethargy, hypotonia, convulsions and mental retardation.

Bank and Morrow (1972) have recently described three brothers having hyperglycinaemia associated with a spinal cord disorder with upper and lower motor neurone signs in the legs. There was no disturbance of the arms or the cranial nerves and sensation and sphincter actions were normal. The mental state was normal and none of the other features of hyperglycinaemia were present. Investigations of the metabolism of these cases showed a defect in the conversion of glycine to serine and this was exacerbated when oral glycine was given. No pathological studies could be made on these patients who remained well apart from their paraparesis.

Subacute Necrotising Encephalomyelopathy (Leigh's Disease)

Under the name subacute necrotising encephalopathy, Leigh (1951) described the clinical findings of necropsy appearances in a 7-month-old infant who presented with a six-week history of immobility, failure to thrive and sweating. The infant was blind, deaf and had spastic limbs with absent tendon reflexes. At necropsy only the brain was abnormal and this showed areas of vascular proliferation affecting the thalamus and neighbouring grey matter around the third ventricle, and the grey matter of the brain stem. In the spinal cord this remarkable vascular proliferation was present in the posterior columns (medial more than lateral) of the cervical and upper thoracic regions.

Leigh suggested, from the similarity of the histological appearances to those of Wernicke's encephalopathy, that a defect of carbohydrate metabolism involving the vitamin B group was present. This appears to be the case from the many subsequent case reports which show raised pyruvate and lactate levels in the blood. In addition acetoacetate, β-hydroxybutyrate and alanine are raised (Crome and Stern, 1972).

Pathology in the Spinal Cord

In addition to the capillary proliferation seen in the spinal cord, as described originally by Leigh, degeneration of posterior, lateral and anterior white columns of the type seen in subacute combined degeneration has been observed. The anterior grey horns show atrophy with neuronal loss and gliosis, and this has been associated with peripheral neuropathy.

REFERENCES

ALAJOUANINE, T., CASTAIGNE, P., CAMBIER, J. and ESCOUROLLE, E. (1967). Maladie de Charcot-Marie. Etude anatomo-clinique d'une observation suivie pendant 65 ans. *Presse méd.*, **75**, 2745–2750.

ANDRE-VAN LEEUWEN, M. (1949). Sur deux cas familiaux de maladie de Friedreich avec atrophie optique précoce globale et grave. *Rev. neurol.*, **81**, 941–956.

BANK, W. J. and MORROW, G. (1972). A familial spinal cord disorder with hyperglycinemia. *Arch. Neurol. (Chic.)*, **27**, 136–144.

BASSEN, F. A. and KORNZWEIG, A. L. (1950). Malformation of erythrocytes in case of atypical retinitis pigmentosa. *Blood*, **5**, 381–387.

BEHAN, W. M. H. and MAIA, M. (1974). Strümpell's familial spastic paraplegia: genetics and neuropathology. *J. Neurol. Neurosurg. Psychiat.*, **37**, 8–20.

BELL, J. M. and CARMICHAEL, E. A. (1939). On hereditary ataxia and spastic paraplegia. *Treas. hum. Inherit.*, **4**, Pt 3, 141–281.

BIEMOND, A. (1928). Neurotische Muskelatrophie und Friedreichsche Tabes in derselben Familie. *Dtsch. Z. Nervenheilk.*, **104**, 113–145.

BROWNELL, D. B., OPPENHEIMER, D. R. and HUGHES, J. T. (1970). The central nervous system in motor neurone disease. *J. Neurol. Neurosurg. psychiat.*, **33**, 338–357.

BYERS, R. K. and BANKER, B. Q. (1961). Infantile muscular atrophy. *Arch. Neurol. (Chic.)*, **5**, 140–164.

CHARCOT, J. M. and JOFFROY, A. (1869). Deux cas d'atrophie musculaire progressive. *Arch. Physiol. norm. path. (Paris)*, **2**, 354–367.

CHARCOT, J. M. and MARIE, P. (1886). Sur une forme particulière d'atrophie musculaire progressive, souvent familiale, débutant par les pieds et les jambes, et atteignant plus tard les mains. *Rev. Méd. (Paris)*, **6**, 97–138.

COLMANT, H. J. (1958). Die myatrophische Lateralsklerose. In *Handbuch der Speziellen Pathologischen Anatomie und Histologie*, Vol.

XIII/2B, pp. 2624–2692. Ed. by W. Scholz. Berlin-Göttingen-Heidelberg: Springer.

CROME, L. and STERN, J. (1972). *Pathology of Mental Retardation*, 2nd edit. Edinburgh: Churchill Livingstone.

DÉJERINE, J. (1883). Étude anatomique et clinique sur la paralysie labio-glosso-laryngée. *Arch. Physiol. norm. path.* (*Paris*), 3.s., **2**, 180–227.

DÉJERINE, J. and ARMAND-DELILLE, P. (1903). Un cas d'atrophie musculaire, type Charcot-Marie, suivi d'autopsie. *Rev. neurol.*, **11**, 1198–1201.

DICK, A. P. and STEVENSON, C. J. (1953). Hereditary spastic paraplegia. Report of a family with associated extrapyramidal signs. *Lancet*, **1**, 921–923.

ESTABLE, C. (1931–1932). Zur histopathologie der Friedreichschen Krankheit nebst einigen Bemerkungen über die Leitungsbahnen des Rückenmarkes. *Trav. Lab. Recher. Biol. Univ. Madrid*, **27**, 1–110.

FRIEDREICH, N. (1873). *Über progressive Muskelatrophie, über wahre und falsche Muskelhypertrophie*. Berlin: Hirschwald.

GOWERS, W. R. (1880). Five cases of locomotor ataxy in members of the same family. *Lancet*, **2**, 618.

GREENFIELD, J. G. (1954). *The Spino-cerebellar Degenerations*. Oxford: Blackwell.

GREENFIELD, J. G. and STERN, R. O. (1927). The anatomical identity of the Werdnig-Hoffmann and Oppenheim forms of infantile muscular atrophy. *Brain*, **50**, 652–686.

HIRANO, A. L. T., KURLAND, L. T. and SAYRE, G. P. (1967). Familial amyotrophic lateral sclerosis. *Arch. Neurol.* (*Chic.*), **16**, 232–243.

HOFFMANN, J. (1893). Ueber chronische spinale Muskelatrophie im Kindesalter, auf familärer Basis. *Dtsch. Z. Nervenheilk.*, **3**, 427–470.

HUGHES, J. T. and BROWNELL, B. (1969). Ultrastructure of muscle in Werdnig-Hoffmann disease. *J. neurol. Sci.*, **8**, 363–379.

HUGHES, J. T. and BROWNELL, B. (1972). Pathology of peroneal muscular atrophy (Charcot-Marie-Tooth disease). *J. Neurol. Neurosurg. Psychiat.*, **35**, 648–657.

HUGHES, J. T., BROWNELL, B. and HEWER, R. L. (1968). The peripheral sensory pathway in Friedreich's ataxia. *Brain*, **91**, 803–818.

HUGHES, J. T. and JERROME, D. (1971). Ultrastructure of anterior horn motor neurones in the Hirano-Kurland-Sayre type of combined neurological system degeneration. *J. neurol. Sci.*, **13**, 389–399.

HUNT, J. R. (1921). Dyssynergia cerebellaris myoclonica. *Brain*, **44**, 490–538.

KURLAND, L. T. (1957). Epidemiologic investigations of amyotrophic lateral sclerosis. III. A genetic interpretation of incidence and geographic distribution. *Proc. Mayo Clin.*, **32**, 449–462.

LAMBRIOR, A. A. (1911). Un cas de maladie de Friedreich avec autopsie. *Rev. neurol.*, **22**, 525–540.

LEIGH, D. (1951). Subacute necrotizing encephalomyelopathy in an infant. *J. Neurol. Neurosurg. Psychiat.*, **14**, 216–221.

MARINESCO, G. (1894). Contribution à l'étude de l'amyotrophie Charcot Marie. *Arch. Méd. exp.*, **6**, 921–965.

MARINESCO, G. (1928). Contribution à l'étude anatomoclinique de l'amyotrophie Charcot-Marie. *Rev. neurol.*, **35**, II, 543–561.

MENDELL, J. R., CHASE, T. N. and ENGEL, W. K. (1971). Amyotrophic lateral sclerosis. A study of central monoamine metabolism and a therapeutic trial of levodopa. *Arch. Neurol.*, **25**, 320–325.

MOTT, F. W. (1907). Case of Friedreich's disease with autopsy and systematic microscopical examination of the nervous system. *Arch. Neurol. Psychiat., Lond.*, **3**, 180–200.

MUNSAT, T. L., WOODS, R., FOWLER, W. and PEARSON, C. M. (1969). Neurogenic muscular atrophy of infancy with prolonged survival. *Brain*, **92**, 9–24.

ROUSSY, G. and LEVY, G. (1926). Sept cas d'une maladie familiale particulière. *Rev. neurol.*, **1**, 427–450.

RUSSELL, D. S. (1946). Myocarditis in Friedreich's ataxia. *J. Path. Bact.*, **58**, 739–748.

SAINTON, P. (1899). *L'Amyotrophie, Type Charcot-Marie.* Paris: G. Steinheil.

SALT, H. B., WOLFF, O. H., LLOYD, J. K., FOSBROOKE, A. S., CAMERON, A. H. and HUBBLE, D. V. (1960). On having no beta-lipoprotein. A syndrome comprising abeta-lipoproteinaemia, acanthocytosis and steatorrhoea. *Lancet*, **2**, 325–329.

SCHWARZ, G. A. (1952). Hereditary (familial) spastic paraplegia. *Arch. Neurol. Psychiat. (Chic.)*, **68**, 655–682.

SCHWARZ, G. A. and LIU, C.-N. (1956). Hereditary (familial) spastic paraplegia. *Arch. Neurol. Psychiat. (Chic.)*, **75**, 144–162.

SMITH, W. E. (1885). Hereditary or degenerative ataxia. *Boston med. surg. J.*, **113**, 361.

SOBREVILLA, L. A., GOODMAN, M. L. and KANE, C. A. (1964). Demyelinating central nervous system disease, macular atrophy and acanthocytosis (Bassen-Kornzweiz syndrome). *Amer. J. Med.*, **37**, 821–828.

SPILLANE, J. D. (1940). Familial pes cavus and absent tendon-jerks: its relationship with Friedreich's disease and peroneal muscular atrophy. *Brain*, **63**, 275–290.

SPILLER, W. G. (1910). Friedreich's ataxia. *J. nerv. ment. Dis.*, **37**, 411–435.

TOOTH, H. H. (1886). *The Peroneal Type of Progressive Muscular Atrophy.* London: Lewis.

TOOTH, H. H. (1887). Recent observations on progressive muscular atrophy. *Brain*, **10**, 243–253.

VIRCHOW, R. (1855). Ein Fall von progressiver Muskelatrophie. *Virchows Arch. path. Anat.*, **8**, 537–540.

WERDNIG, G. (1891). Zwei frühinfantile hereditäre Fälle von progressiver Muskelatrophic unter dem Bilde der Dystrophie, ober auf neurotischer Grundlage. *Arch. Psychiat. Nervenkr.*, **22**, 437–480. (Reprinted as a translation in *Arch. Neurol.*, **25** (1971), 276–278.)

CHAPTER IV

VASCULAR DISORDERS

ANATOMICAL CONSIDERATIONS

The spinal cord has one of the most complex blood supplies of any part of the body and it is necessary to understand some of its complexity before discussing the problem of its vascular disorders. Early studies on this subject are those of Ross (1880), Adamkiewicz (1882), and Kadyi (1886). More recent studies are those of Tureen (1936), Suh and Alexander (1939), Herren and Alexander (1939), Bolton (1939), Krogh (1945), Yoss (1950), Corbin (1961), Jellinger (1966), Neumayer (1967), and Piscol (1972).

The following account is based upon the reports of these authors amplified by personal observations from anatomical dissections and injection studies of the spinal cord vascular systems (Hughes, 1967).

The major named arteries of the body concerned with spinal cord blood supply are the following:

(I)	Vertebral	⎫
	Ascending cervical (inferior thyroid)	⎬ arising from
	Deep cervical (costocervical trunk)	subclavian
	Superior intercostal (costocervical trunk)	⎭ artery
(II)	Intercostal	⎱ arising from
	Lumbar	⎰ aorta
(III)	Iliolumbar	⎱ arising from inter-
	Lateral sacral	⎰ nal iliac arteries

From above downwards, in respect to the region of the spinal cord supplied, these are the vertebral, the ascending cervical branch of the inferior thyroid and the deep cervical and superior intercostal branches of the costocervical trunk. All these arteries arise from the subclavian artery and supply the spinal cord throughout its cervical region and also the upper two thoracic spinal cord segments. The remainder of the thoracic cord is supplied by intercostal branches of the aorta whilst the lumbosacral cord is supplied by the analogous lumbar aortic branches and the iliolumbar and lateral sacral arteries arising from the internal iliacs. All these arteries give rise to spinal branches which enter the intervertebral foramina and after entering the dural sheath divide into anterior and posterior branches which accompany the anterior and posterior nerve roots respectively. In this way there are paired radicular tributaries to the three major spinal cord arteries, the anterior spinal and the right and left posterior spinal arteries. These three longitudinally oriented arteries are the basis of the arterial supply of the spinal cord. The anterior spinal artery, which is by far the most important, commences by the union of the anterior spinal branches given off within the cranial cavity from each vertebral artery, and passes down the spinal cord in or near the anterior median sulcus. It receives the paired tributaries already mentioned but most of these are small and the blood supply is mainly dependent on four to ten of these arterial tributaries which are especially large. The number, laterality and segmental position of these major tributaries is quite variable but at least one joins the cervical cord, two the thoracic and one the lumbar cord. The posterior spinal arteries (right and left) are smaller than the anterior spinal artery; each begins as an intracranial branch of the vertebral artery and proceeds down the spinal cord in the posterior lateral sulcus receiving tributaries accompanying each posterior nerve root. In contrast to the few major tributaries to the anterior spinal artery the posterior spinal arteries receive from 30–40 well developed radicular tributaries though none are of comparable size to the large major tributaries to the anterior spinal artery. Anastomosis occurs between the anterior and posterior spinal arteries at their caudal portions around the cauda equina. There is very little anastomosis between the anterior and posterior spinal arteries at each spinal cord segment occurring by circumferential anastomoses passing round the spinal cord.

We now must consider the detailed vascular supply of a single spinal cord segment. From the anterior spinal artery a sulcal artery is given off into the anterior median sulcus, this passes backwards and then usually turns either left or right to enter the spinal cord. In the lumbar and sacral regions some of these divide into left and right branches but the more usual arrangement is to turn into one side of the cord only. The sulcal arteries are most numerous in the lumbar region and fewest in the thoracic region where there may be only one per cord segment. These sulcal arteries with their branches supply the anterior and lateral grey horns, the central grey matter and Clarke's column, that is, all the grey matter save the posterior horn. They also supply the bulk of the white matter of the anterior and lateral columns with the exception of a peripheral rim supplied by coronal branches. These coronal branches arise from the anterior spinal artery and form a meningeal plexus passing laterally around the cord and meeting, but forming an imperfect anastomosis with the posterior spinal branches. In this manner the anterior two-thirds of the spinal cord segment is fed from the anterior spinal artery. The remaining third, comprising the posterior white columns and the posterior horn is supplied by the two posterior spinal arteries through small penetrating branches, the largest of which accompany the posterior nerve roots.

The venous drainage of the spinal cord mainly corresponds to the arterial supply. The differences are that there are more venous tributaries both within and around the cord and also of large size in the intervertebral foramina. These major venous trunks are variable and frequently duplicated, although posteriorly there is a single median spinal vein corresponding in importance to the two posterior spinal arteries. Anastomosis of the spinal veins is freer than that of the arteries and whilst the territorial division into a posterior third and anterior two-thirds is maintained, the boundaries do not appear to be so immutable.

In this complicated pattern of spinal cord blood supply, one can pick out some features of especial importance in the understanding of vascular disorders of the spinal cord.

(i) The multiplicity of feeding sources into the spinal arterial system. This forms a powerful reserve of arterial supply secure except by interruption at specially vulnerable places.

(ii) The dependence on a small number of tributary arteries of inconstant position which are relatively so large that the numerous other tributaries may be interrupted with impunity.

(iii) The strict division into anterior and posterior spinal artery territories which supply two-thirds and one-third of the cross-sectional area respectively.

(iv) The absence of significant anastomosis between anterior and posterior spinal arteries circumferentially around the cord. The anterior spinal artery at the cauda equina does make a good anastomosis with the lower part of the posterior spinal arteries.

(v) The overwhelming importance in the whole system of the single (usually) anterior spinal artery.

(vi) The reserve of venous drainage so that venous obstruction rarely damages the spinal cord.

PATHOLOGICAL OBSERVATIONS

The concept of a syndrome of spinal-cord infarction dates from Bastian (1886) who, in his book, wrote:

> "Thus one of the common causes of ordinary degenerative or ischaemic softening as it occurs in the encephalon, is undoubtedly operative in the cord, and I must, therefore, express my strong dissent from the statement made by Charcot (*Localisation*, p. 41) to the effect that 'softening secondary to arterial obstruction, whether it be due to thrombosis or to embolism, are almost unknown accidents in the spinal cord'."

In defence of Charcot it must be said that clinical accounts of such cases are still infrequent and necropsy reports remain particularly rare. Some idea of this is given by the report of Blackwood (1958) who reviewed the 3,737 necropsies performed at the National Hospital for Nervous Diseases, London during the 50 year period 1909–58. He found only nine cases of vascular disorder affecting the spinal cord. Five were instances of acute infarction from cervical disc disease (three cases), trauma (one case), and dissecting aneurysm (one case). The four chronic cases were cases of sub-acute necrotic myelitis which Blackwood then classified as spinal thrombophlebitis. My own interest in this subject gathered 26 cases from the department of neuropathology at Oxford over a 20-year period. These cases have been described elsewhere (Hughes, 1965), when the possible sites (Fig. 22) of obstruction to the vascular supply of the spinal cord were grouped under seven headings:

Aorta (Subclavian)
Vertebral arteries
Intercostals (Lumbar arteries)
Radicular tributaries
Anterior and posterior spinal arteries
Small spinal arteries
Veins

Aortic Cases

Aortic atheroma is very common but it is rare for the clinical worker to attribute spinal cord ischaemia to this cause. The report of Hughes and Brownell (1966) describes cases in which severe

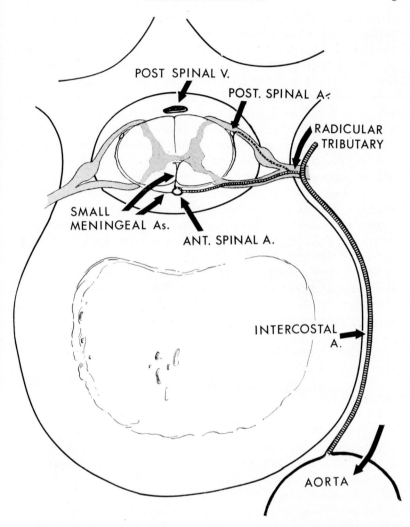

FIG. 22.—Diagram showing arrangement of the blood supply to the spinal cord. The arrows indicate the possible sites of vascular obstruction: aorta, intercostal artery, radicular tributary, anterior and posterior spinal arteries, small spinal arteries, veins.

aortic atheroma had caused ischaemic damage to the spinal cord, the clinical course being an ill-defined chronic paraparesis. This condition is probably more common than is realised, for without necropsy the diagnosis is difficult. Skinhøj (1954) diagnosed, on clinical grounds, this condition in three cases.

The commonest aortic cause of acute spinal cord ischaemia is probably dissecting aneurysm, in which dissection of the tunica media by a haematoma compresses the origins of the intercostal or lumbar arteries. The clinical signs of neurological involvement are often slight and the scrutiny of the spinal cord then shows only trivial findings. But when an important intercostal or lumbar artery is blocked extensive spinal cord infarction can occur, although published necropsy reports are few. Thompson (1956) reviewed seven previous cases adding his own where dissection had blocked the right fifth and left sixth and seventh intercostal arteries, causing infarction from T5 to T12 spinal cord segments. A similar state of spinal cord infarction can occur in aortic trauma (Hughes, 1964a). In this case a tear in the aortic wall caused a mural haematoma which compressed the 2nd–5th intercostal arteries at their origin. The spinal cord was infarcted from T3 to T7 spinal segments.

Spinal cord infarction rarely is caused by aortic thrombosis (Dragescu and Petrescu, 1929; Corbin, 1961) but only if the upper abdominal aorta is occluded. Aortic occlusion during modern surgical manoeuvres has been responsible for many cases which have been well documented. Adams and van Geertruyden (1956) were able to analyse twenty-four instances of ischaemia of the spinal cord due to aortic surgery (Fig. 23). From the data of these cases they were able to conclude that when the aorta is occluded below the origin of the renal arteries the spinal cord does not suffer ischaemia, although ischaemic efforts on roots or peripheral nerves may occur. When the aortic occlusion is suprarenal then spinal cord damage may occur, depending, in any individual case, on the type of segmental pattern of the spinal cord blood supply.

Vascular disturbance of the spinal cord can occur in the "adult" type of coarctation of the aorta in which the narrowing of the aorta is confined to a small segment usually beyond the origin of the subclavian artery. Coarctation of the aorta is not common and Fawcett (1905) in reviewing 22,316 necropsies at Guy's Hospital between 1826 and 1902 found only 18 cases. The proportion of cases with a spinal cord complication is very small. Woltman and Shelden (1927) in reviewing the world literature found 32 cases with neurological complications and these formed 7 per cent of the reports studied by them. Most of these reports were of cerebral complications such as intracerebral or subarachnoid haemorrhage.

The complications affecting the spinal cord are fewer and are of two types:

1. *Those due to a reduced blood supply to the caudal part of the spinal cord.*

These complications formed the majority of the observations reported by Tyler and Clark (1958). The paresis, sensory impairment and sphincteric disturbance were attributed in these cases to

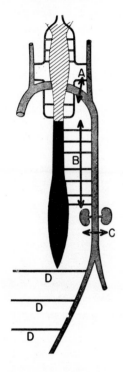

FIG. 23.—This diagram illustrates the potential neurological damage which may follow aortic occlusion.

A. Suprarenal occlusion of the aorta interferes with the circulation of both the spinal cord and peripheral nerves.

B. Occlusion of the intercostal arteries interferes with only the blood supply of the spinal cord.

C. Infrarenal occlusion of the aorta interferes only with the circulation to the peripheral nerves through arteries D.

ischaemia and hypotension of the part of the spinal cord normally supplied by arteries derived from the aorta beyond the constriction.

2. *Complications due to the hypertension present in the body in arteries derived proximal to the aortic constriction.*

This second group includes cases in which enlarged collateral vessels have caused compression of the spinal cord. There have been no necropsy reports of cases of coarctation in which a local hypertension caused a spinal cord syndrome but this suggestion was made in a case studied clinically by Weenink and Smilde (1964).

Vertebral Artery Cases

The unique situation of the vertebral arteries merits their separate consideration. These arteries ascend in the vertebral foramina of the transverse processes of the upper six cervical vertebrae. In this part of their course they may be affected by atheromatous narrowing and occasionally involved by tumour, but these chronic and unilateral processes do not usually impair the spinal cord blood supply. Thrombosis is rare and usually affects the origin of the artery as in the case of Boudin *et al.* (1959). The main hazard to the intraspinal part of the vertebral arteries is trauma, for by this one or both arteries may be suddenly obstructed. In two cases (Hughes, 1964b) the trauma to the cervical spine had torn the C5–6 intervertebral disc and both vertebrals were compressed (Figs. 24 and 25). In both cases

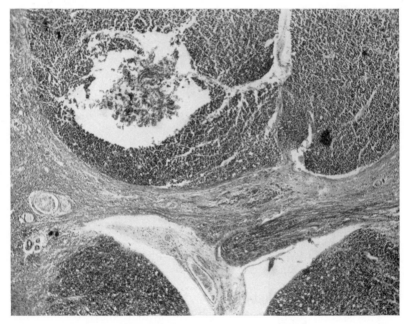

Fig. 24.—Acute infarction. Photomicrograph of a histological section through the spinal cord at C4 segmental level showing the cephalic limit of the infarcted "cone" as a round area of necrosis in the right posterior column. Case of cervical spine trauma with obstruction to the vertebral arteries. Weil ×30.

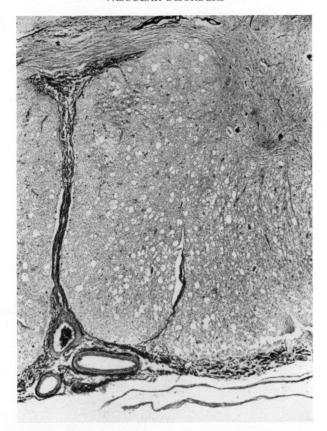

FIG. 25.—Chronic ischaemia. Low-power view showing the anterior median sulcus, grey commissure, anterior horn and anterior white column. The white matter shows spongy myelin and fibre loss (worst centrally), whilst the grey matter of the anterior horn shows gliosis with depletion of neurones. Case of intermittent obstruction of the vertebral arteries. Holmes × 30.

necropsy showed that infarction of the lower cervical region of the spinal cord had occurred.

Intercostal and Lumbar Artery Cases

This group consists of the rare cases in which the paired aortic branches, such as the intercostal and lumbar arteries, are involved. Such cases have most frequently resulted from surgical operations. Thoracoplasty (Rouques and Passelecq, 1957) and pneumonectomy (Binet, quoted by Corbin, 1961) have occasionally been responsible, but the majority of cases have been caused by a sympathectomy. Hughes and MacIntyre (1963) reviewed other reported cases whilst adding the clinical and necropsy findings in a case following thoracolumbar sympathectomy. At necropsy the spinal cord from T6 to L1 was shrunken, the anterior part of the cord being affected (Fig. 26). Examination of the radicular arteries showed large vessels accompanying left C3, right C8, left

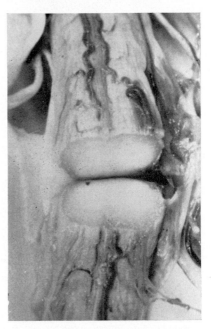

FIG. 26.—Anterior aspect of the spinal cord showing also the appearance displayed by a transverse slice. The anterior part of the spinal cord is shrunken from atrophy and appears grey on cut section. Case of infarction following thoraco-lumbar sympathectomy.

T1, then a big gap until left L2. Hence there was no major tributary to the anterior spinal artery between T1 and L2 segments. The missing vessel in all probability was the right T9 tributary since, during the operation of right thoracolumbar sympathectomy, the right ninth rib was resected.

Radicular Tributary Cases

The group of cases, in which arterial obstruction has occurred in the intervertebral foramina, is mostly made up of advanced malignant disease of the spine. In these cases the spinal canal is normal but the cord is infarcted by a mass of malignant tumour which obstructs the radicular tributaries by infiltrating the intervertebral foramina. Spiller (1925) described two such cases due to carcinomatous infiltration and demonstrated the ischaemic mechanism by autopsy studies. I have seen several cases of this nature (Hughes, 1965). Psoas abscess due to tuberculous osteitis can operate in a similar manner and in my experience extensive infarctions can occur without any tuberculous exudate within the spinal canal. Very rarely a similar sequence of pathological events can be encountered in herpes zoster. It is not generally realised that the lesion of herpes zoster looks histologically like an infarct in the posterior root ganglion, and also that there is in this disease a tendency to thrombosis. When the affected posterior root ganglion has an accompanying important radicular tributary, then extensive spinal cord infarction may occur as in the case described in Chapter VI.

Anterior Spinal Artery Occlusion

The clinical syndrome of anterior spinal artery occlusion was first recognised in life by Spiller (1909) and the correctness of his diagnosis was demonstrated at autopsy. The upper portion of the anterior spinal artery was affected and the cord damage extended from the fourth cervical to the third thoracic segments. Spiller called the disorder syphilitic acute anterior poliomyelitis and for some time the condition was regarded as being caused by syphilitic disease (Chung, 1926). Recent cases are not often due to syphilis and in a review of the literature, Hughes and Brownell (1964) found cases due to atheroma, trauma, coarctation of aorta, aortic occlusion, haemangioma of the spinal cord, infection, and bleeding into a neurofibroma (affecting a radicular artery). In our own case reported in this paper we attributed the thrombosis of the anterior spinal artery to an effect of coexisting cervical spondylosis.

Clinical findings in anterior spinal artery occlusion.—The clinical course of this condition is dramatic and characteristic. In the space of a few minutes there is onset of pain in the back and dysaesthesiae and weakness of the hands and arms. In a few hours the condition has progressed to a flaccid areflexic paresis of the upper limbs with dissociated anaesthesia. The lower limbs develop a spastic paraparesis and there is paralysis of bladder and bowel. The cerebrospinal fluid is usually normal. The neurological deterioration then ceases and the usual progression is to a considerable degree of recovery except for the lower motor neurone lesion affecting the arms which is permanent.

Pathological findings in anterior spinal artery occlusion.—The spinal cord at necropsy shows softening due to acute infarction which involves its anterior part. The exact boundary between the anterior infarcted area and the posterior preserved tissue is well demarcated but varies from case to case. This variability may be

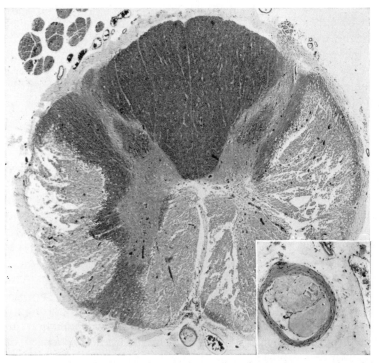

FIG. 27.—Anterior spinal artery thrombosis. Myelin stained transverse section of the spinal cord at T12 segmental level. There is acute infarction of the anterior parts of the cord due to thrombosis of the anterior spinal artery. Weil × 7.

The inset shows an enlarged picture of the thrombus in the anterior spinal artery Haematoxylin and Van Gieson × 28.

caused by the extent of the spinal artery thrombosis which may involve small sulcal and even intramedullary vessels, Hughes and Brownell (1964). The region of infarction is roughly symmetrical and always involves both anterior horns and the grey commissure (Fig. 27). The anterior white columns are usually completely infarcted but the extent of involvement of the lateral columns varies. The microscopical appearances are those of necrosis with abundant lipid phagocytes. The grey matter shows profound ischaemic damage with no surviving neurones in the infarcted area. At a later stage the spinal cord shows severe shrinkage of the affected area due to the loss of both nervous and glial elements. The glial scar that results, although striking in appearance, is merely the proliferation of the processes of those fibrous astrocytes at the margin of the infarct which were not destroyed by the ischaemia.

Posterior Spinal Artery Occlusion

Occlusion of one or both of the posterior spinal arteries is rarely recognised clinically and there have been very few clinicopathological reports (Williamson, 1895). Hughes (1970) reported the clinical course and necropsy findings in one case and reviewed nine other reported cases.

The neurological syndrome was similar in the reviewed cases and the differences were due to the varying extent of the infarcted region of the spinal cord. Onset with pain or dysaesthesia is common but paresis or paralysis of the lower limbs and trunk rapidly supervene. The bladder and bowel are usually paralysed. This description refers to the period immediately following the onset of the neurological syndrome when there is a cord transection caused mainly by swelling and oedema. If the patient survives this period then considerable neurological improvement may occur.

The cause of the posterior spinal artery occlusion has only rarely been ascertained. In earlier cases syphilitic arteritis has been suspected. In one case indirect trauma was the cause and in another embolisation of atheromatous cholesterol material. In the case seen by the author (Hughes, 1970) the cause was an intrathecal injection of phenol given to treat severe intractable pain due to a carcinoma of the oesophagus. The nature of the infarction is unremarkable but its extent is very variable. Very elaborate search for the arterial occlusion or occlusions is required and in some reports no thrombosis or other occlusive pathology was found.

Small Spinal Arteries

Involvement of small arteries occurs in a diverse group of diseases. Cases in which the small arteries of the spinal cord are affected are infrequent, but the group contains some interesting pathological entities. Formerly meningovascular syphilis accounted for many cases but this disease is now rare at least in a severe form. In my experience severe endarteritis is now more common in tuberculous meningitis and I have examined several cases in which the ischaemic damage to the cord was severe. These two infective diseases are dealt with in Chapter VI along with a similar state produced by sarcoidosis.

Periarteritis nodosa.—This disorder, classified among the collagen diseases, is characterised by a widespread arteritis which may inflict serious ischaemic damage on the central and peripheral nervous systems. Malamud and Foster (1942) in their experience found that the central nervous system was involved in about 20 per cent of cases, but the spinal cord was only involved seriously in 2 per cent of cases. Other reports with necropsy accounts of spinal cord damage are those of Boyd (1940), Roger et al. (1953), and Haft et al. (1957). For a full review of periarteritis nodosa affecting the nervous system the reader is referred to Walthard and Walthard (1957). The histological appearance of periarteritis nodosa is too well known to be detailed here. The small meningeal arteries are affected with obliteration, thrombosis, and occasionally haemorrhage. The damage to the spinal cord is infarction caused by obliteration of the small arteries.

Embolism.—In cases of bacterial endocarditis it is usually possible at necropsy to find microscopical evidence of bacterial embolism to the spinal cord, but these small lesions have not been vocal clinically. It is much rarer to encounter serious infarction caused by larger emboli, and these, perhaps, do not readily enter the circuitous arterial supply of the spinal cord. Among the few reports of this kind is that of Harrington (1925). Madow and Alpers (1949) suggested embolism as an explanation of their case in which spinal-cord infarction had followed cardiac infarction.

Embolism of portions of atheromatous plaques from the aorta was described in two cases by Wolman and Bradshaw (1967) and this type of lesion was produced experimentally in dogs and monkeys by Finlayson, Mersereau and Moore (1972). Venous embolism will be described later. The embolism of fibrocartilage (Fig. 28a and b) from the nucleus pulposus into the anterior spinal artery and into spinal veins was described by Hubert et al. (1974) who review other instances of this strange phenomenon.

Caisson Disease

Air embolism of the spinal cord occasionally follows some surgical procedure such as pneumothorax (Wickler et al., 1937),

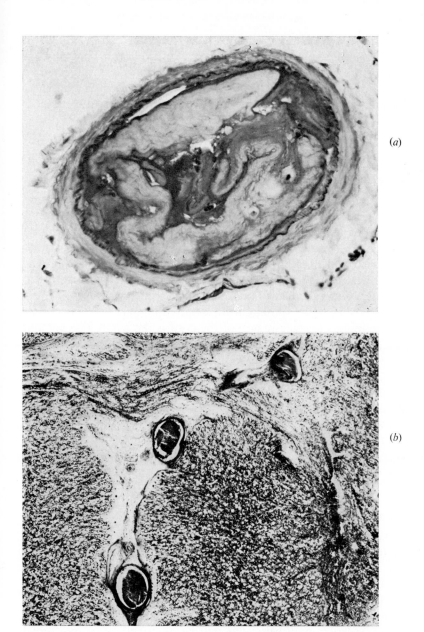

(a)

(b)

Fig. 28.—Case of Hubert *et al.* (1974). (a) Anterior spinal artery occluded by fibro-cartilage. Masson's trichrome ×43. (b) Veins of the anterior spinal system occluded by fibrocartilaginous material. Haematoxylin and eosin ×270.

but the greatest number of cases result from the condition known as decompression sickness (Haymaker, 1957). This disease formerly occurred only in divers and other workers subjected to high air pressure in underwater caissons (hence caisson disease) or similar pressurised containers. High-altitude aviation presents a similar hazard of rapid decompression to subatmospheric pressures. The symptoms appear shortly after rapid lowering of the barometric pressure to which the individual has become adjusted. Obese individuals are more susceptible; this was known in 1868 by Mericourt for sponge divers, confirmed in 1908 by Boycott and Damant for caisson workers and is well recognised in aviation decompressions (Haymaker, 1957). The cause of the disorder is the appearance of gaseous nitrogen bubbles in the tissues, blood vessels and even the cerebrospinal fluid. These gaseous bubbles embolise, but many are trapped and absorbed in the lungs. The damage sustained by the spinal cord is probably due to nitrogen bubbles arising locally (autochthonous) and this preferential involvement of the spinal cord is of great interest.

The upper thoracic region of the cord is the worst affected and the brain may escape entirely. Within the cord the ischaemic lesions occur almost exclusively in the white matter. Although any part of the white columns may be involved there are favoured locations such as the centre of each posterior column, a site of predilection reminiscent of multiple sclerosis. Spinal cord involvement predominates in caisson disease with little cerebral involvement. The situation is reversed in the high-altitude decompression cases where the brain is often seriously involved by large ischaemic lesions and the spinal cord may escape serious damage.

Veins

Acute venous infarction.—The concept of a spinal cord syndrome of venous infarction produced by obstruction of the veins draining the spinal cord is not new and the literature of the subject is detailed elsewhere (Hughes, 1971). These cases are frequently confused with cases of vascular malformation of the spinal cord complicated by thrombosis of some of the abnormal vessels. These vascular malformations will be described later and here I shall discuss only the occlusion of veins which were hitherto normal. The world literature contains only a handful of well-documented cases and the account which follows is based on seven reported cases of thrombosis and one of embolism (Hughes, 1971).

The clinical story is remarkably consistent. The onset is rapid and invariably with pain which may affect the back, legs or abdomen. Within one or two days weakness and loss of sensation in the legs and trunk appear often combined with paralysis of the bladder and bowel. The number of cells and the level of protein in the spinal fluid may be raised but these changes may be slight or absent. Myelography has shown moderate swelling of the spinal cord with a partial holdup of the Myodil column. The illness in all the cases has rapidly progressed and the outcome has been death in the first or second week of the neurological illness. The bad prognosis in the reviewed cases was due mainly to the gravity of the associated disease which caused the venous infarction of the spinal cord. The condition is almost impossible to diagnose during life and so the actual prognosis may be better. We cannot know how many cases evade detection.

The pathology of the condition has so seldom been described that the following case report (Hughes, 1971) is given in some detail.

CASE REPORT

A 67-year-old man, a retired civil servant previously in good health, began to complain of pain in the bottom of his spine radiating to the lumbar region and the lowermost ribs. After three days, this pain disappeared but by then he had the feeling of "pins and needles" in his left leg, which the following day became weak. He now had retention of urine and soon developed weakness in the right leg. On admission to hospital, one week after his first symptom of pain, he had a complete areflexic flaccid paraplegia of both lower limbs with loss of all sensation below the level of the sixth thoracic dermatome. He had retention of urine and paralysis of the bowel. On the day of admission, a lumbar puncture produced clear spinal fluid under a pressure of 90 mm of CSF and manometric responses were normal. There were 5 lymphocytes per mm^3, and the protein was 15 mg per 100 ml. A myelogram showed a free flow of iofendylate (Myodil) up to the skull when the patient was prone, but in the supine position there was slight obstruction at the level of the fourth thoracic vertebral body. On the day after admission, he developed a complete left hemiplegia with a corresponding sensory loss on the left side. A right carotid angiogram showed a complete occlusion of the right internal carotid artery. He died the following day, having survived his paraplegic neurological syndrome for eight days.

General necropsy findings.—The immediate cause of death was extensive pulmonary infarction due to emboli from thrombosed leg and pelvic veins. The pancreas, which weighed 142 g, was abnormal in that the neck of the organ was expanded by a whitish tumour which histologically had the structure of an adenocarcinoma. The heart weighed 380 g. The aorta showed only a trace of atheroma near the bifurcation. The orifices of the intercostal and lumbar spinal arteries were examined and found to be patent. The right internal carotid artery contained recent ante-mortem thrombus extending from its origin to its termination. The inferior vena cava contained portions of ante-mortem thrombus as did both common iliac veins. Ante-mortem thrombus was also present in both femoral veins and in the small leg veins draining into them. The left saphenous vein was completely filled with ante-mortem thrombus.

The brain, which weighed 1,510 g, showed extensive recent infarction in the territory of the right middle cerebral artery and related to the obstruction by thrombus of the right internal carotid artery. The spine was fixed with the spinal cord *in situ*, and after fixation, the spinal canal was opened by a posterior laminectomy. When the spinal cord and the spinal meninges were removed, the extradural spinal veins inside the spinal canal from the mid-thoracic region downward were grossly enlarged into a plexus of huge venous channels, most of which contained ante-mortem thrombus.

Examination of spinal cord.—Externally, the spinal cord, the spinal vessels, and the leptomeninges were normal above the mid-thoracic region. From this area downward, the leptomeninges were opaque and thickened, the spinal veins were prominent, and the spinal cord was swollen (Fig. 29). The anterior spinal artery could be identified as far as the mid-thoracic region, but from about T-10 downward it was completely concealed by the prominence of the anterior spinal vein. The anterior spinal artery, received major tributaries accompanying left C-5, right C-6, left T-3, right T-7, and left T-9 anterior nerve roots. No major tributaries could be identified caudal to this. The veins of the lower half of the spinal cord from T-9 downward were distended both anteriorly and posteriorly (Fig. 29). The main draining veins accompanied right T-10, left T-10, right T-11, and left L-1 posterior nerve roots and these were greatly distended (Fig. 29). Transverse cuts (Fig. 30) across the spinal cord showed a normal appearance down to the C-8 segment. In the upper part of the T-1 segment, there was blood-staining affecting the posterior columns, and by examining in transverse slices down the T-1 segment, the blood-staining was seen to enlarge into a central blood clot about 1 mm in diameter. This blood clot grew down to T-6 where it was a 6 × 4 mm oval area consisting entirely of blood clot with a surrounding margin of blood-staining. Throughout the T-7 segment, the picture changed to haemorrhagic infarction involving all but a peripheral rim of spinal cord. The extent of the infarction increased, and at T-10, T-11, and T-12 segments, the whole cross-sectional area of the spinal cord was involved. Throughout the L-1 segment, the area of infarction diminished, and at the L-2 segment, only the posterior columns were involved in haemorrhagic infarction. The infarction

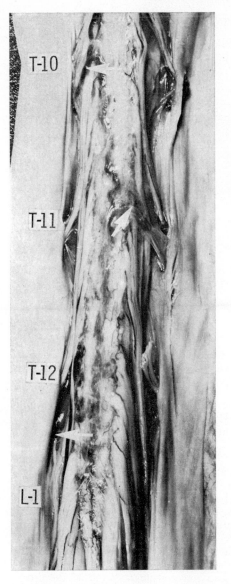

ACUTE VENOUS INFARCTION

FIG. 29.—Spinal cord from T-10 to L-3 viewed from the posterior aspect with the dura mater opened. The spinal cord is swollen and there is intense congestion. The posterior spinal veins are greatly distended as are the major venous tributaries (arrows) accompanying the left T-10, right T-11, and left L-1 posterior nerve roots. The figures identify the spinal nerve roots. Enlargement is twice normal size.

ended in the L-4 segment as a small dark-red area in the posterior columns. The sacral segments were normal.

Histological examination.—Transverse sections were taken at the following segmental levels: C-4, C-7, C-8, T-1 to T-12, L-1 to L-5, S-1, and S-3 to S-5. Paraffin sections were stained by haematoxylin

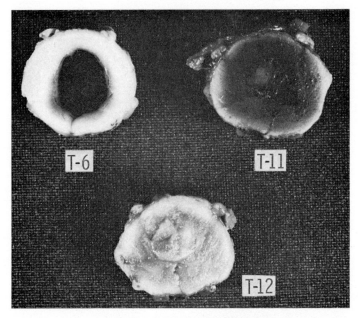

ACUTE VENOUS INFARCTION

FIG. 30.—Transverse slices at three levels of the spinal cord viewed from the caudal aspect. At T-6 (top left), there is a large oval haematoma situated centrally. At T-11, there is haemorrhagic infarction which is less intense at T-12. Enlargement is three times normal size.

and eosin, haematoxylin and Van Gieson, Nissl, Weil, and Holmes stains for nerve axons (Fig. 31).

(1) *C-4, C-7 and C-8.*—The only abnormality in these segments was early Wallerian degeneration in the posterior white columns seen at high magnification as early breakdown of myelin and axonic material seen in the appropriate stained sections.

(2) *T-1 to T-12 and L-1 to L-3.*—A state of haemorrhagic infarction affected every one of these 15 consecutive spinal cord segments. The area of the infarction and the position and extent of the haematoma, described macroscopically, are illustrated in Fig. 31. The infarction was of the type seen in venous obstruction and differed in the following ways from arterial infarction: The infarction was extremely haemorrhagic and associated with a large haematoma (Fig. 32). The extent of the infarction (15 consecutive segments) and of the cross-sectional area of the cord affected was much greater than that seen in arterial infarction. The necrosis of the grey and white matter was less complete and the margin of the infarcted region less distinct than seen in arterial infarction of the spinal cord. The site of the venous obstruction was sought in these sections but clearly the primary pathology lay outside the spinal cord. All the spinal veins and the

tributary radicular veins were dilated, but none of these vessels near the spinal cord were found to be obstructed.

(3) *L-5, S-1 and S-3 to S-5.*—The only abnormality in these spinal cord segments was early Wallerian degeneration seen in the cortico-spinal tracts.

In this case the cause of the extensive venous thrombosis was a thrombotic state associated with a carcinoma of the body of the pancreas.

Chronic Venous Obstruction

Most of the reports that can be accepted as cases of spinal thrombophlebitis are those with acute venous infarction (*see above*). Other cases with venous thrombosis are more likely to be examples of arteriovenous communication in which there may be thrombosis of some of the abnormal vessels. It is probable that the cases of Foix and Alajouanine (1926), Bodechtel and Erbslöh (1957), Greenfield and Turner (1939), Antoni (1952) and of Mair and Folkerts (1953) were of this type which we shall now consider.

Arteriovenous aneurysm of the spinal cord.—Antoni (1962) reported five cases, in which myelomalacia had been caused, he believed, by arteriovenous shunting of blood through a venous fistula. In my experience (Hughes, 1967) this is the commonest type of angiomatous condition of the spinal cord although in many cases it is difficult to demonstrate the actual arteriovenous communication. Many of the cases reviewed in the monograph of Wyburn-Mason (1944) were of this type.

The clinical course is that of a progressive paresis and sensory disturbance affecting first the lower and then the upper limbs. The disorder frequently spans many years but there may be acute exacerbations, sometimes with subarachnoid bleeding. No signifi-cant pathology has been described outside the spinal cord. The spinal leptomeninges are opaque due to fibrous thickening. The spinal vessels are the key to the condition. In my experience, there is usually a slightly enlarged but otherwise normal arterial system with normal radicular tributaries to the anterior spinal artery. The venous drainage is enlarged, being tortuous with many very dilated veins, but it is usually possible to make out a completely arranged venous system abnormal only due to dilatation. Super-imposed on all the normal vessels is an abnormal group of large varicosities which, when followed, are seen to form one large convoluted venous channel (Fig. 33). The histology of this abnormal vessel is that of an expanded vein thickened by mural connective tissue proliferation but lacking any proper muscular coat.

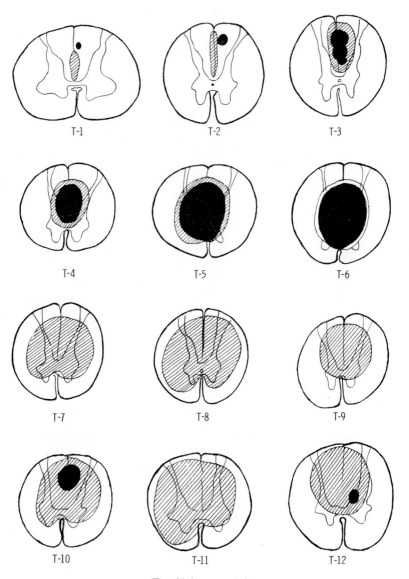

FIG. 31 (*see opposite*).

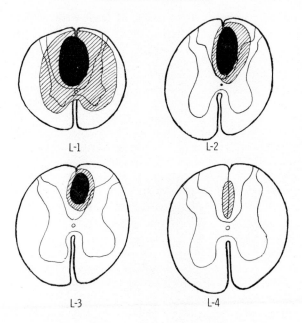

ACUTE VENOUS INFARCTION

FIG. 31.—Drawings from camera lucida tracings of transverse sections of the spinal cord at 12 segmental levels. The shaded area indicates haemorrhagic infarction (*see* Fig. 30), whilst the black area indicates haematoma (*see* Figs. 30 and 32).

These vessels were called "arterialised veins" by Cushing and Bailey (1928) and "fistulous veins" by Antoni (1962). The spinal cord itself is atrophied because of necrosis and loss of grey and white matter (Fig. 34). There are sometimes large abnormal vessels inside the cord but they are far fewer than the surplus leptomeningeal vessels. The necrosis has given rise to many lipid phagocytes and many new capillaries have formed, often with surrounding connective tissue proliferation.

Cavernous haemangioma of the spinal cord.—Vascular hamartomas occur in the spinal cord as in other structures and they have several features distinguishing them from the arteriovenous aneurysms. A most significant finding is their association with angiomas of other structures such as brain, kidney, and pancreas (Willis, 1962). It is often difficult to separate the reports of cavernous haemangiomas from haemangioblastomas, and sometimes the two coexist.

The clinical course of these cases, at least with respect to their spinal cord anomalies, is often a silent period before the sudden onset of symptoms due to haemorrhage. Haemorrhage may be

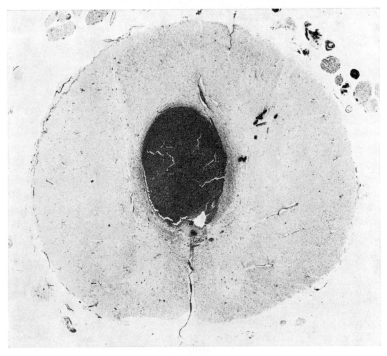

ACUTE VENOUS INFARCTION

FIG. 32.—Photomicrograph of a transverse section of the spinal cord at T-4 segmental level. The spinal cord is swollen and congested. The black oval central lesion is a haematoma. Haematoxylin and Van Gieson × 10.

subarachnoid or intramedullary and these cases are the commonest cause, save trauma, of haematomyelia. The situation in the spinal cord differs from both the types previously described. The spinal cord throughout much of its extent appears normal. The only abnormality of the arterial and venous system is that they are more extensive and capacious than normal. The region where the haemangioma lies is swollen and discoloured. On transverse slicing there is a circumscribed spherical mass very similar to a comparable cavernous haemangioma of the liver. The sections show this lesion to be made up of large vascular spaces and of thin-walled irregular channels. Around and in the malformation there may be haemosiderin deposition and a terminal haemorrhage may have contributed to death. Calcification is sometimes present in these lesions both in the vessel walls and as free masses in the tissues. The arterial supply and venous drainage of these masses is greater than normal for the situation, but there is none of the massive leptomeningeal venous plexus seen in the other two types. It is possible that an intramedullary lesion of this nature may in itself constitute an arteriovenous fistula, but I have never seen a case of this nature.

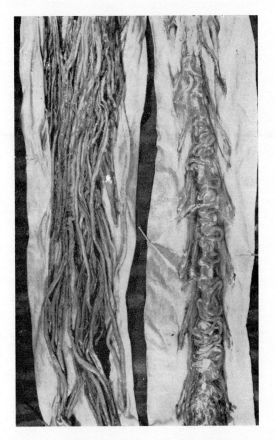

FIG. 33.—Case of Foix-Alajouanine disease. The picture illustrates the posterior aspect of the spinal cord (divided into upper and lower portions). The thoracic cord (on right) shows an enormous dilated convoluted vessel on its posterior aspect. Note how on the nerve roots of the cauda equina (on left) all the radicular venous tributaries are dilated.

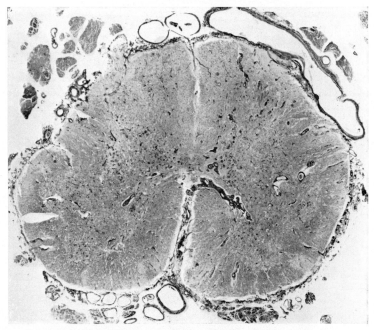

FIG. 34.—Transverse section through the sacral region of the spinal cord of the case in Fig. 33. There are many abnormal small vessels inside the spinal cord. Note that with one exception there are anterior and posterior spinal arteries and spinal veins which are normal apart from moderate dilatation. The exception is the single large abnormal vessel on the postero-lateral aspect of the spinal cord. Weil × 7.

REFERENCES

ANATOMICAL REPORTS

ADAMKIEWICZ, A. (1882). Die Blutgefässe des menschlichen Rücken-markes. II. Teil. Die Gefässe der Rückenmarks oberfläche. *S.-B. Akad. Wiss. Wien, Kl. Abt. III*, **85**, 101–130.

BOLTON, B. (1939). Blood supply of human spinal cord. *J. Neurol. Psychiat.*, **2**, 137–148.

CORBIN, J. L. (1961). *Anatomie et Pathologie Artérielles de la Moelle.* Paris: Masson.

HERREN, R. Y. and ALEXANDER, L. (1939). Sulcal and intrinsic blood vessels of human spinal cord. *Arch. Neurol. Psychiat. (Chic.)*, **41**, 678–687.

HUGHES, J. T. (1967). *The blood supply and vascular disorders of the human spinal cord.* D.Phil. thesis. University of Oxford.

JELLINGER, K. (1966). *Zur Orthologie und Pathologie der Rückenmarks-durchblutung.* Wien: Springer.

KADYI, H. (1886). Über die Blutgefässe des menchlichen Rückenmarkes. *Anat. Anz.*, **1**, 304–314.

KROGH, E. (1945). Studies on the blood supply to certain regions in the lumbar part of the spinal cord. *Acta physiol. scand.*, **10**, 271–281.

NEUMAYER, E. (1967). *Die vasculäre Myelopathie.* Wien: Springer.

PISCOL, K. (1972). *Die Blutversorgung des Rückenmarkes und ihre klinische Relevanz.* Berlin: Springer.

ROSS, J. (1880). Distribution of the arteries of the spinal cord. *Brain*, **3**, 80–84.

SUH, T. H. and ALEXANDER, L. (1939). Vascular system of human spinal cord. *Arch. Neurol. Psychiat. (Chic.)*, **41**, 659–677.

TUREEN, L. L. (1936). Effect of experimental temporary vascular occlusion on the spinal cord. I. Correlation between structure and functional changes. *Arch. Neurol. Psychiat. (Chic.)*, **35**, 789–807.

YOSS, R. E. (1950). Vascular supply of the spinal cord: The production of vascular syndromes. *Univ. Mich. med. Bull.*, **16**, 333–345.

PATHOLOGICAL REPORTS

ADAMS, H. D. and VAN GEERTRUYDEN, H. H. (1956). Neurologic complications of aortic surgery. *Ann. Surg.*, **144**, 574–610.

ANTONI, N. (1952). Myelitis periphlebitica or angioma racemosum venosum medullae spinalis. *Proc. Int. Congr. Neuropath. Rome*, **3**, 557–564.

ANTONI, N. (1962). Spinal vascular malformations (angiomas) and myelomalacia. *Neurology (Minneap.)*, **12**, 795–804.

BASTIAN, H. C. (1886). *Paralyses, Cerebral, Bulbar and Spinal.* London: H. K. Lewis.

BLACKWOOD, W. (1958). *In* Discussion on vascular disease of the spinal cord. *Proc. roy. Soc. Med.*, **51**, 543–547.

BODECHTEL, G. and ERBSLÖH, F. (1957). Die Foix-Alajouaninesche Krankheit. In *Handbuch der Speziellen Pathologischen Anatomie und Histologie*, Vol. XIII/IB, pp. 1576–1599, Ed. by W. Scholz. Berlin-Göttingen-Heidelberg: Springer.

BOUDIN, G., PÉPIN, B., BARBIZET, J. and LABRAM, C. (1959). Syndrome de l'hémimoelle gauche par thrombose de la portion initiale de l'artere vertébrale chez un sujet porteur d'une thrombose ancienne de la sous-clavière gauche. *Bull. Soc. méd. Hôp. Paris*, **75**, 164–170.

BOYD, L. J. (1940). Periarteritis nodosa. IV. Neuromyositic manifestations. *Bull. N.Y. med. Coll.*, **3**, 272–279.

CHUNG, M. F. (1926). Thrombosis of spinal vessels in sudden syphilitic paraplegia. *Arch. Neurol. Psychiat. (Chic.)*, **16**, 761–771.

CORBIN, J. L. (1961). *Anatomie et Pathologie Artérielles de la Moelle.* Paris: Masson.

CUSHING, H. and BAILEY, P. (1928). *Tumours arising from the blood vessels of the brain. Angiomatous malformations and haemangioblastomas.* Springfield, Ill.: Charles Thomas.

DRAGESCU, R. and PETRESCU, M. (1929). Contribution à l'étude de la pathogènie de la paraplegie consécutive a la thrombose aortique. *Bull. Soc. méd. Hôp. Buc.*, **11**, 243–248.

FAWCETT, J. (1905). Coarctation of the aorta as illustrated by cases from the post-mortem records of Guy's Hospital from 1826 to 1902. *Guy's Hosp. Rep.*, **59**, 1–19.

FINLAYSON, M. H., MERSEREAU, W. A. and MOORE, S. (1972). Spinal cord emboli in dogs and monkeys and their relevance to aortic atheroma in man. *J. Neuropath. exp. Neurol.*, **31**, 535–547.

FOIX, C. and ALAJOUANINE, T. (1926). La myélite necrotique subaigüe. *Rev. neurol.*, **2**, 1–42.

GREENFIELD, J. G. and TURNER, J. W. A. (1939). Acute and subacute necrotic myelitis. *Brain*, **62**, 227–252.

HAFT, H., FINNESON, B. E., CRAMER, H. and FIOL, R. (1957). Periarteritis nodosa as a source of subarachnoid haemorrhage and spinal cord compression. *J. Neurosurg.*, **14**, 608–616.

HARRINGTON, A. W. (1925). Embolism of the spinal cord. *Glasg. med. J.*, **103**, 28–32.

HAYMAKER, W. (1957). Decompression sickness. In *Handbuch der Speziellen Pathologischen Anatomie und Histologie*, Vol. XIII/IB, pp. 1600–1672. Ed. by W. Scholz. Berlin-Göttingen-Heidelberg: Springer.

HUBERT, J.-P., ECTORS, M., KETELBANT-BALASSE, P. and FLAMENT-DURAND, J. (1974). Fibrocartilaginous venous and arterial emboli from the *nucleus pulposus* in the anterior spinal system. *Europ. Neurol.*, **11**, 164–171.

HUGHES, J. T. (1964a). Spinal-cord infarction due to aortic trauma. *Brit. med. J.*, **2**, 356.

HUGHES, J. T. (1964b). Vertebral artery insufficiency in acute cervical spine trauma. *Int. J. Paraplegia*, **1**, 1–14.

HUGHES, J. T. (1965). Vascular disorders of the spinal cord. *Int. J. Paraplegia*, **2**, 207–213.

HUGHES, J. T. (1967). *The Blood Supply and Vascular Disorders of the Human Spinal Cord.* D.Phil. thesis, University of Oxford.

HUGHES, J. T. (1970). Thrombosis of the posterior spinal arteries. *Neurology (Minneap.)*, **20**, 659–664.

HUGHES, J. T. (1971). Venous infarction of the spinal cord. *Neurology (Minneap.)*, **21**, 794–800.

HUGHES, J. T. and BROWNELL, B. (1964). Cervical spondylosis complicated by anterior spinal artery thrombosis. *Neurology (Minneap.)*, **14**, 1073–1077.

HUGHES, J. T. and BROWNELL, B. (1966). Spinal cord ischaemia due to arteriosclerosis. *Arch. Neurol. (Chic.)*, **15**, 189–202.

HUGHES, J. T. and MACINTYRE, A. G. (1963). Spinal cord infarction occurring during thoraco-lumbar sympathectomy. *J. Neurol. Neurosurg. Psychiat.*, **26**, 418–421.

MADOW, L. and ALPERS, B. J. (1949). Involvement of the spinal cord in occlusion of the coronary vessels. *Arch. Neurol. Psychiat. (Chic.)*, **61**, 430–440.

MAIR, W. G. P. and FOLKERTS, J. F. (1953). Necrosis of the spinal cord due to thrombophlebitis (subacute necrotic myelitis). *Brain*, **76**, 563–575.

MALAMUD, N. and FOSTER, D. B. (1942). Periarteritis nodosa. A clinicopathologic report, with special references to the central nervous system. *Arch. Neurol. Psychiat. (Chic.)*, **47**, 828–838.

ROGER, H., POURSINES, Y. and ROGER, J. (1953). La périartérite nodueuse (maladie de Kussmaul), ses manifestations neurologiques. *Ann. Méd.*, **54**, 22–50.

ROUQUES, L. and PASSELECQ, A. (1957). Syndrome de Brown-Séquard après thoracoplastie. *Rev. neurol.*, **97**, 146–147.

SKINHØJ, E. (1954). Arteriosclerosis of spinal cord: 3 cases of pure "syndrome of anterior spinal artery". *Acta psychiat. scand.*, **29**, 139–144.

SPILLER, W. G. (1909). Thrombosis of the cervical anterior median spinal artery: syphilitic acute anterior poliomyelitis. *J. nerv. ment. Dis.*, **36**, 601–613.

SPILLER, W. G. (1925). Rapidly developing paraplegia associated with carcinoma. *Arch. Neurol. Psychiat. (Chic.)*, **13**, 471–478.

THOMPSON, G. B. (1956). Dissecting aortic aneurysm with infarction of spinal cord. *Brain*, **79**, 111–118.

TYLER, H. R. and CLARK, D. B. (1958). Neurological complications in patients with coarctation of aorta. *Neurology (Minneap.)*, **8**, 712–718.

WALTHARD, B. and WALTHARD, K. M. (1957). Periarteritis nodosa. In *Handbuch der Speziellen Pathologischen Anatomie und Histologie*, Vol. XIII/1B, pp. 1563–1575. Ed. by W. Scholz. Berlin-Göttingen-Heidelberg: Springer.

WEENINK, H. R. and SMILDE, J. (1964). Spinal cord lesions due to coarctatio aortae. *Psychiat. Neurol. Neurochir.* (Amst.), **67**, 259–269.

WIKLER, A., MARMOR, J. and HURST, A. (1937). Air embolism of the spinal cord following attempted pneumothorax. *J. Amer. med. Ass.*, **108**, 403–431.

WILLIAMSON, R. T. (1895). Spinal softening limited to the parts supplied by the posterior arterial system of the cord. *Lancet*, **2**, 520–522.

WILLIS, R. A. (1962). *The Borderland of Embryology and Pathology*, 2nd edit. London: Butterworth.

WOLMAN, L. and BRADSHAW, P. (1967). Spinal cord embolism. *J. Neurol. Neurosurg. Psychiat.*, **30**, 446–454.

WOLTMAN, H. W. and SHELDEN, W. D. (1927). Neurologic complications associated with congenital stenosis of isthmus of aorta; case of cerebral aneurysm with rupture and case of intermittent lameness presumably related to stenosis of isthmus. *Arch. Neurol. Psychiat. (Chic.)*, **17**, 303–316.

WYBURN-MASON, R. (1944). *The Vascular Abnormalities and Tumours of the Spinal Cord and its Membranes*. London: Henry Kimpton.

CHAPTER V

TRAUMA TO THE SPINAL CORD

"One having a dislocation in a vertebra of his neck while he is unconscious of his two legs and his two arms, and his urine dribbles. An ailment not to be treated."
Case 31. *The Edwin Smith Surgical Papyrus, c.* 3000–2500 B.C.

The above translation, given by Breasted (1930), is from the *Edwin Smith Surgical Papyrus*, an interesting document dating from the time of the building of the Great Pyramid of Gizeh. Injuries to the spinal cord must have been well known to this ancient surgical author for the case quoted is one of several recorded in the papyrus. In many other early records there is evidence of interest in the clinical syndrome which was known to Hippocrates, Celsus, Ambrose Pare and Paulus of Aegina. In more recent times the subject has excited especial interest in the study of war casualties. The subject is referred to in connection with the American Civil War (Otis, 1870), but the first spate of reports deal with spinal injuries sustained in the First World War. The British casualties were described by Holmes (1915) and their pathological aspects detailed by Buzzard and Greenfield (1921). French contributions are those of Claude and Lhermitte (1914–15) and Roussy and Lhermitte (1918), whilst Foerster (1929) reported cases occurring in the German Army. In World War II injuries to the spinal cord received a great deal of attention. The experience gained from British cases was reported by Guttmann (1953) who at Stoke Mandeville in England introduced measures of treatment and rehabilitation (Guttmann, 1973) that have made his National Spinal Injuries Unit a model for the rest of the world. Important American reports are those of Pool (1945) and Haynes (1946). The story of spinal cord injuries in warfare has been brought up to date for the Korean conflict by Boshes *et al.* (1954) and for the war in Vietnam by Jacobs and Berg (1971) and by Heyl (1972). Meanwhile civilian spinal cord injuries have increased in numbers. Originally mining accidents predominated but today the speed of modern transport gives to an accident the degree of trauma hitherto seen commonly only on the battlefield. Wolman (1964) and Hughes (1974) have reviewed the pathology of this subject.

Here we shall list certain types of injuries that recur in these reports.

Gross Spinal Trauma

Gun-shot wounds, the high-velocity missiles concerned in war casualties (Fig. 35), and the trauma of modern civilian accidents make this group a large one. The damage to the spinal column is complex with comminuted fractures which are often combined with dislocations and result in an unstable or malaligned spinal canal. The spinal cord may be directly damaged by a missile or

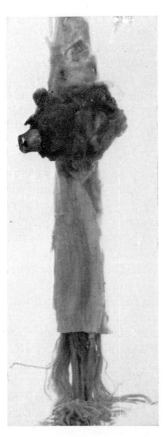

contused by displaced bone fragments. Tissue oedema and haemorrhage add compressive forces which cause further damage to the spinal cord; later secondary infection may occur. In this group the damage sustained by the spinal cord is maximal; it very often amounts to a complete cord transection and may affect the cord over a considerable length involving several consecutive spinal cord segments.

Discrete Penetrating Wounds

This type of discrete lesion of the spinal cord is a feature of stab wounds which are usually made with a knife, although other weapons have frequently been recorded (Lipschitz and Block, 1962). These discrete lesions have attracted interest because of the anatomical studies they permit; Brown-Séquard's account in 1868 (Greenfield and Russell, 1963) is perhaps the most famous, but many others have used such opportunities to advantage. There are interesting papers on stab wounds by Petrén (1910), Rand and Patterson (1929), and St. John and Rand (1953).

FIG. 35.—Anterior aspect of spinal cord (within the dura mater) of a British soldier wounded by a bullet at Normandy in June, 1944.

The spinal laminae prevent a knife from entering directly from behind, consequently the direction of the wound is such that the weapon enters the spinal canal slightly lateral of the midline. Because of this, hemisection of the spinal cord is common, either one lateral half of the cord being severed or sometimes there is damage to both posterior columns. The damage reported to the spinal cord ranges from a small localised lesion to a complete transection. Usually there is little bleeding and only slight associated damage, but there are exceptions when an important vessel is severed.

Flexion, Rotational, Compressive and Extension Injuries

The way in which trauma injures the spine is often complex but certain patterns of spinal and spinal-cord injury recur and merit separate description.

Flexion injuries.—Sudden forcible flexion of the spine (usually the cervical region) causes a wedge compression fracture of the vertebral bodies. Often there is accompanying dislocation which may be bilateral and is associated with tearing of the capsular ligaments and of the longitudinal ligament. Often one or more articular processes fracture, the consequence being a fracture–dislocation. The upper spine tends to move forward with relation to the portion of spine below the injury. This malalignment narrows the spinal canal and the spinal cord is pinched between the lower vertebral body and the neural arch of the vertebra above.

The type of neck injury caused by judicial hanging is of this nature and an accidental fracture of this type is sometimes called a "Hangman's fracture" (Schneider *et al.*, 1965).

Rotational injuries.—Rotational forces are frequently combined with forcible flexion of the spine, again usually in the cervical region. The result is often a unilateral fracture–dislocation with rotational displacement of the two separated portions of the spinal canal. The spinal canal may later appear undeformed but the spinal cord has been damaged by the displacement permitted at the time of injury by the fracture–dislocation.

Compression injuries.—Compression fractures may occur in the cervical region but are most often seen in the thoracolumbar region (Yashon and White, 1974). Here the articular facets are deep and strong, and so are less likely to fracture. The violence is borne by the vertebral body which may burst shooting bone fragments and disc material into the spinal canal. In this way we may see spinal cord compression of sudden onset at the time of the injury.

Extension injuries.—Extension injuries affecting the spinal cord differ appreciably in their clinical presentation from those already described. The hyperextension, usually from a forward fall, causes spinal cord damage mainly in elderly persons with cervical spondylosis. There may be tearing of an intervertebral disc and angulation of the spinal cord already narrowed by cervical spondylosis. This type of injury has occurred from quite modest force, and hyperextension during general anaesthesia is a particular hazard. The necropsy findings in three cases of this type were described by Hughes and Brownell (1963*a*).

Birth injuries.—Kennedy (1836) and Parrot (1869) were the first authors to describe obstetrical trauma to the spinal cord. Important reports are those of Crothers (1923), of Ford (1925), and there are reviews with added case reports by Crothers and Putnam (1927), Stern and Rand (1959) and Leventhal (1960). The most recent review is that of Byers and Bresnan (1974). In all these accounts breech extraction of the child predominates though it is possible to have spinal cord damage with a head presentation.

In the fetus at term the spine consists of soft cartilage and is only feebly supported by the toneless neck muscles. The dura mater is probably the strongest structure, and in necropsy experiments traction will lengthen the spinal column up to two inches yet the stretched dura mater does not tear. It is probable that in these cases of birth injury during breech extraction there is traction and hyperextension of the cervical spine sufficient to tear the dura. Such dural tears have been found in the necropsies which often show vertebral injury. The spinal cord may be torn and is often compressed by haematoma either extradural or subdural in situation.

This complication of obstetrical trauma is probably commoner than would be suggested by the number of published reports. The remedy is the more careful management of breech presentations. In breech extraction the prevention of perinatal asphyxia is usually emphasised, and for this reason a rapid second stage of labour is desirable. This requirement of a rapid breech extraction is the cause of applying grossly unphysiological force to the newborn neck.

The modern trend for delivery of breech presentations by Caesarean section will avoid this particular obstetric hazard.

Pathological Findings following Spinal-cord Trauma

The extent of the damage seen at necropsy depends on the type of injury, but the histological appearances vary strikingly according to the period of survival. For this reason I shall consider the pathological findings under the headings, early, intermediate and late changes. Some of the terms currently used require definition. *Concussion*, used in the sense of a reversible physiological disturbance of spinal cord function caused by sudden jarring of the spine, is a valuable term for an interesting phenomenon analogous to cerebral concussion. For obvious reasons, the histopathology of the human condition has not been investigated. In experimental studies (Wagner *et al.*, 1971) it is clear that minor reversible changes of blood supply occur.

Contusion (L. *contundere*, to crush) means a crushing injury to the spinal cord and this may range in severity from a trivial lesion to one in which the cord is pulped. Contusion is more common than a complete tear through the spinal cord. *Haematorrhachis* means haemorrhage into the spinal canal; the blood may be in the extradural, subdural or subarachnoid spaces. *Haematomyelia* means a definite collection of blood in the spinal cord and should not be confused with the more common haemorrhagic pulping seen in severe contusion.

Early pathological changes (Fig. 36).—The immediate consequences of a spinal-cord contusion or tear are damaged or severed nerve fibres, effects on neurone cell bodies, and exudative phenomena.

The nerve fibres undergo swelling and distintegration of both axonic material and of myelin. The axons when mildly damaged show beading; a more severe state is a line of droplets of axonic material in the former position of the axon, whilst in grossly contused specimens one demonstrates with appropriate methods only a silver-impregnated dust of displaced axonic fragments. The point where an axon is completely torn may develop a terminal swelling called an end-bulb. The myelin tubes show corresponding changes ranging from a bubbly appearance in the myelin, only detected under high-power magnification, to complete fragmentation of the myelin giving abundant fatty droplets scattered amid the axonic material. The cell bodies of the neurones show either disruption or axonal reaction (central chromatolysis), the latter state occurring when damage remote from the cell body affects it by the severance of its axon.

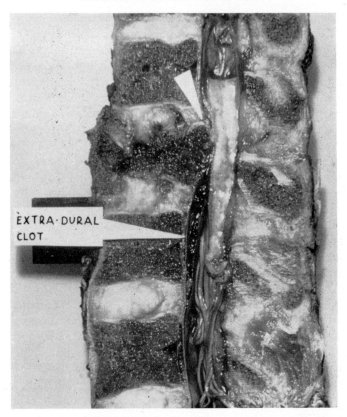

EXTRA-DURAL
CLOT

FIG. 36.—Sagittally sawn specimen of spine from a case of trauma involving the spinal cord. Note the gross compressive fracture of a vertebral body and the extra-dural blood clot in the spinal canal. Appearances soon after injury.

The exudative changes are oedema, red-cell diapedesis, and an inflammatory reaction of polymorphs, lymphocytes and plasma cells. These changes are best sought (Fig. 37a, b) a little distance from the main site of injury where they are obscured by the haemorrhage and haemorrhagic necrosis caused directly. Oedema, when slight, may be perivascular but often the oedematous state affects the whole cross-sectional area of the cord. As in the cerebrum, it is seen microscopically as rounded perivascular spaces in the white matter and perineuronal spaces in the grey matter. All these changes cause swelling of the spinal cord which becomes rounded and tense within the leptomeninges and dura, the subarachnoid and subdural spaces being obliterated. In

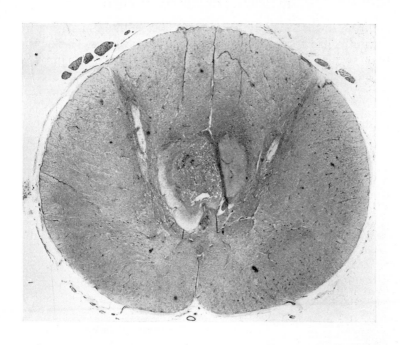

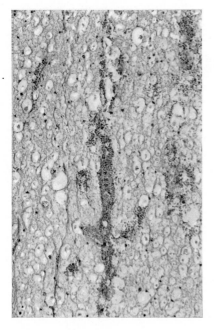

Fig. 37a (above).—Transverse section of the spinal cord at C5 segmental level from a case of acute trauma. The picture shows the situation above the main damage with a 'core' of damaged spinal cord in the posterior columns. Appearance two days after injury. Haematoxylin and eosin × 8.

Fig. 37b (left).—Oedema and red cell diapedesis due to injury. Same case as in Fig. 37a. Haematoxylin and eosin × 60.

addition to the swelling there is purple discoloration arising from the initial haemorrhage and later from venous stasis. This oedematous swollen state of the acutely damaged cord has provoked much speculation. It is clear that this cord swelling enlarges the region of traumatic damage and the final form is often in the shape of a spindle. This comprises a fusiform region of cord softening affecting one or more segments and ending above and below by tapering to end as a small round area often situated in

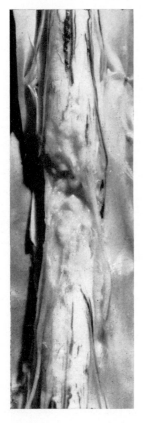

FIG. 38.—Anterior aspect of the spinal cord (with dura opened and reflected) from a case of trauma involving the spinal cord. Note the softened state of the destroyed part of the cord. Appearance ten days after injury.

the posterior columns. This round area has often been commented upon and is probably a core of damaged tissue forced up by pressure. The appearances may be exaggerated by post-mortem handling which also may push softened material into the dural root sleeves.

Measures in the immediate post-traumatic period to combat this cord swelling have frequently been advocated, but the majority opinion favours conservative measures. Decompression by laminectomy and the opening of the dura is very hazardous and violent extrusion of a considerable amount of softened cord has resulted.

Apart from the oedema the exudative phenomena are the diapedesis of red cells and the appearance of leucocytes. The red cell extravasation, when marked, forms petechial haemorrhages; this feature, together with hyperaemia due to vascular dilatation, is attributable to venous stasis, an accompaniment of the swollen state of the cord. The cellular reaction is at first polymorphonuclear but later lymphocytes predominate.

For an account of the appearances in experimental trauma to the spinal cord the reader is referred to Wagner *et al.* (1971). The ultrastructural changes are described in Dohrmann *et al.* (1971).

Intermediate pathological changes (Fig. 38).—The changes described above cover the state of the injured cord in the immediate post-traumatic period. After two or three weeks these acute changes subside and are gradually replaced by a reparative phase of long duration, up to two or more years. The pathological changes in this phase are so different from those in the early and late stages that they merit separate description.

The oedema has now largely subsided and the smaller haemorrhages have been absorbed. The larger haemorrhages form cysts and these, if of any considerable longitudinal extent, have the form of a syrinx. The occasional development of a progressive syringomyelia will be described later. The polymorphs of the acute reaction are replaced by lymphocytes and large macrophages. The most striking cell everywhere is the lipid phagocyte or compound granular corpuscle. These phagocytes are present wherever necrosis has destroyed nerve fibres and liberated breakdown products. The phagocytes are frequently clustered around small vessels forming rosette-like aggregates. In grossly damaged areas there are countless closely apposed lipid phagocytes; where the damage was slight, as in the margins of the injury, then scattered fat granule cells are present. The presence of astrocytic gliosis in any particular part of the lesion depends on the degree of damage; where this is slight, there is a reactive astrocytosis. In the severely damaged areas the glia has perished along with the parenchyma, and here organisation is by young fibroblasts. The neuronal changes now seen are only a few examples of central chromatolysis (axonal reaction); these persist with their swollen cytoplasm and eccentric nuclei for some time.

Late pathological changes (Fig. 39).—Gradually the pathological picture just described changes and when the survival period is 5–10 years or more then a different situation is found at necropsy. There is now a traumatic scar with acellular collagenous connective tissue uniting meninges to the spinal canal and to the spinal cord and in this connective tissue scar anatomical planes are often indistinct.

The histological features are well seen in the Van Gieson stain. The grossly damaged regions of the cord are replaced by connective tissue occupying the position of the former blood clot and the severe parenchymal necrosis. The less damaged regions of the cord and always a margin above and below the main damage show an intense astrocytic fibrous gliosis. The mossy glial network with occasional astrocyte cell bodies replaces the damaged

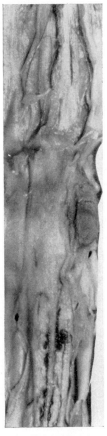

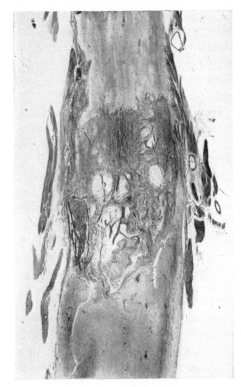

Fig. 40

Fig. 39

Fig. 39.—Anterior aspect of spinal cord (with dura opened and reflected) showing late appearance of a traumatic lesion. Above and below, the spinal cord can be made out, but in the region of the injury a connective tissue scar replaces the damaged spinal cord and blends with the thickened dura mater. Appearances 12 years after injury.

Fig. 40.—Longitudinal section through the traumatic scar of a case with long survival after a spinal-cord injury. The injured spinal-cord segments are telescoped and three occupy the normal space of one. The centre of the scar is connective tissue which is invaded by regenerating nerve fibres from the posterior roots. Appearances 16 years after injury.

nerve fibres and neurone cell bodies. An interesting regenerative phenomenon is frequently seen in these traumatic scars. The cell bodies of the posterior root ganglia regenerate their central processes into the region of the connective tissue scar. These fibres, which are myelinated but clothed with Schwann-like cells, ramify in the connective tissue in the manner of an amputation neuroma of peripheral nerve (Fig. 40). They do not enter the glial scar nor enter intact nervous tissue. The significance of this phenomenon was reviewed in the report by Hughes and Brownell (1963b) and by Hughes (1974).

Traumatic Syringomyelia

We have mentioned earlier that a longitudinal cavity in the form of a syrinx commonly forms in the intermediate stage of a severe injury to the spinal cord. This cavity replaces the zone of haemorrhagic necrosis seen in the acute stage of the injury and later comes to have a glial and connective tissue lining which sometimes forms a thick wall. The interest in this common feature of spinal cord trauma is that occasionally a post-traumatic syringomyelia develops. (Cossa, 1943; Freeman, 1959; Jung, 1960; Schott et al.,1962, Martin and Maury, 1964; Riffat and Domenach, 1964; Bischof and Nittner, 1965; Barnett et al., 1966; Rossier et al., 1968; Nurick et al., 1970).

Long after the initial injury and at a time when the neurological state has been stable for several months there are signs of an upward extent of the spinal cord lesion. This development can progress rapidly and with an ascent of the neurological signs to reach the medulla. The central part of the spinal cord is the most affected, with neurological signs and myelographic appearances as seen in idiopathic syringomyelia. Whilst in the majority of cases the syringomyelia is an upward cavitation from the original trauma, downward cavitation can occur but is clinically silent because of the existing cord lesion above. In a case I have examined pathologically a combination of upward and downward syringomyelia extending from the trauma was found.

The exact mechanism of these post-traumatic syringes has not been ascertained. In cases I have examined there is a strong suspicion of a communication between the syrinx and the subarachnoid space laterally near a posterior root entry zone.

REFERENCES

BARNETT, H. J. M., BOTTERELL, E. H., JOUSSE, A. T. and WYNN-JONES, M. (1966). Progressive myelopathy as a sequel to traumatic paraplegia. Brain, 89, 159–174.

BISCHOF, W. and NITTNER, K. (1965). Zur Klinik und Pathogenese der vaskulär bedingten Myelomalazien. *Neurochirurgia (Stuttg.)*, **8**, 215–231.

BOSHES, B., ZIVINN, I. and TIGAY, E. A. (1954). Recent methods of management of spinal cord and cauda equina injuries. Comparative study of World War II and Korean experiences. *Neurology (Minneap.)*, **4**, 690–704.

BREASTED, J. H. (1930). *The Edwin Smith Surgical Papyrus*, Vol. 1, p. 327. Chicago: Univ. of Chicago Press.

BUZZARD, E. F. and GREENFIELD, J. G. (1921). *Pathology of the Nervous System*, p. 88. London: Constable.

BYERS, R. K. and BRESNAN, M. J. (1974). Birth injuries of the spinal cord. In *Brock's Injuries of the Brain and Spinal Cord*, 5th edit. Ed. by E. H. Feiring. New York: Springer.

CLAUDE, H. and LHERMITTE, J. (1914–15). Étude clinique et anatomo-pathologique de la commotion médullaire direct par projectiles de guerre. *Ann. Med.*, **2**, 479–506.

COSSA, P. (1943). Syringomyelie secondaire à une blessure de la moelle dorsale supérieure. *Rev. neurol.*, **75**, 39–40.

CROTHERS, B. (1923). Injury of spinal cord in breech extraction as important cause of fetal death and of paraplegia in childhood. *Amer. J. med. Sci.*, **165**, 94–110.

CROTHERS, B. and PUTNAM, M. C. (1927). Obstetrical injuries of spinal cord. *Medicine (Baltimore)*, **6**, 41–126.

DOHRMANN, G. J., WAGNER, F. C., JR. and BUCY, P. C. (1971). The microvasculature in transitory traumatic paraplegia. An electron microscopic study in the monkey. *J. Neurosurg.*, **35**, 263–271.

FOERSTER, O. (1929). *Handbuch der Neurologie Ergänzungsband.* Berlin: Springer.

FORD, F. R. (1925). Breech delivery in its possible relations to injury of the spinal cord, with special reference to infantile paraplegia. *Arch. Neurol. Psychiat. (Chic.)*, **14**, 742–750.

FREEMAN, L. W. (1959). Ascending spinal paralysis. Case presentation. *J. Neurosurg.*, **16**, 120–122.

GREENFIELD, J. G. and RUSSELL, D. S. (1963). Traumatic lesions of the central and peripheral nervous systems. In *Greenfield's Neuropathology*. 2nd edit. Ed. by W. Blackwood, W. H. McMenemy, A. Meyer, R. M. Norman and D. S. Russell. London: Edward Arnold.

GUTTMANN, L. (1953). *British History of the Second World War*. Vol. Surgery. London: H.M.S.O.

GUTTMANN, Sir L. (1973). *Spinal Cord Injuries*. Oxford: Blackwell.

HAYNES, W. G. (1946). Acute war wounds of spinal cord; analysis of 184 cases. *Amer. J. Surg.*, **72**, 424–433.

HEYL, H. L. (1972). Federal programs for the care and study of spinal cord injuries. *J. Neurosurg.*, **36**, 379–385.

HOLMES, G. (1915). The Goulstonian lectures on spinal injuries of warfare. *Brit. med. J.*, **2**, 769–774.

HUGHES, J. T. (1974). Pathology of spinal cord damage in spinal injuries. In *Brock's Injuries of the Brain and Spinal Cord*. 5th edit. Ed. by E. H. Feiring. New York: Springer.

HUGHES, J. T. and BROWNELL, B. (1963*a*). Spinal-cord damage from hyperextension injury in cervical spondylosis. *Lancet*, **1**, 687–690.

HUGHES, J. T. and BROWNELL, B. (1963*b*). Aberrant nerve fibres within the spinal cord. *J. Neurol. Neurosurg. Psychiat.*, **26**, 528–534.

JACOBS, G. B. and BERG, R. A. (1971). The treatment of acute spinal cord injuries in a war zone. *J. Neurosurg.*, **34**, 164–167.

JUNG, E. (1960). Syringomyelie in Kombination mit Entwicklungsstörung der Nieren und mit schwerer Wirbelsäulenverletzung. *Med. Klin.*, **55**, 1678–1679.

KENNEDY, E. (1836). Observations on cerebral and spinal apoplexy, paralysis and convulsions of new-born infants. *Dublin J. med. Sci.*, **10**, 419–444.

LEVENTHAL, H. R. (1960). Birth injuries of the spinal cord. *J. Pediat.*, **56**, 447–453.

LIPSCHITZ, R. and BLOCK, J. (1962). Stab wounds of the spinal cord. *Lancet*, **2**, 169–172.

MARTIN, C. and MAURY, M. (1964). Syndrome syringomyelique apres paraplégie traumatique. A propos de six cas de syndrome syringomyélique cervical survenant dans des paraplégies dorsale ou lombaire. *Presse. med.*, **72**, 2839–2842.

NURICK, S., RUSSELL, J. A. and DECK, M. D. F. (1970). Cystic degeneration of the spinal cord following spinal cord injury. *Brain*, **93**, 211–222.

OTIS, A. (1870). *Medical and Surgical History of the War of the Rebellion* (1861–1865), Vol. 2, part 1, p. 452. Washington D.C.: U.S. Govt. Printing Office.

PARROT, J. (1869). Note sur un cas de rupture de la moelle chez un nouveau-né par suite de manoevres pendant l'accouchement. *Bull. Soc. méd. Hôp. Paris* (2nd series), **6**, 38–45.

PETREN, K. (1910). Ueber die Bahnen der Sensibilität im Ruckenmarke, besonders nach den Fällen von Stichverletzung Studiert. *Arch. Psychiat. Nervenkr.*, **47**, 495–557.

POOL, J. L. (1945). Gunshot wounds of spine; observations from evacuation hospital. *Surg. Gynec. Obstet.*, **81**, 617–622.

RAND, C. W. and PATTERSON, G. H. (1929). Stab wounds of spinal cord; report of 7 cases. *Surg. Gynec. Obstet.*, **48**, 652–661.

RIFFAT, G. and DOMENACH, J. (1964). Syndrome syringo-myélique succédont à un traumatisme médullaire ancien. *Lyon Méd.*, **212,** 1043.

ROSSIER, A. B., WERNER, A., WILDI, E. and BERNEY, J. (1968). Contribution to the study of late cervical syringomyelia syndromes after dorsal or lumbar traumatic paraplegia. *J. Neurol. Neurosurg. Psychiat.*, **31,** 99–105.

ROUSSY, J. and LHERMITTE, J. (1918). *Blessures de la moelle et de la queue de cheval.* Paris: Masson.

ST. JOHN, J. R. and RAND, C. W. (1953). Stab wounds of spinal cord. *Bull. Los Angeles neurol. Soc.*, **18,** 1–24.

SCHNEIDER, R. C., LIVINGSTONE, K. E., CARE, A. J. E. and HAMILTON, G. (1965). "Hangman's fracture" of the cervical spine. *J. Neurosurg.*, **22,** 141–154.

SCHOTT, B., TRILLET, M., VAUTERIN, C. and KOSHBIN (1962). Syndromes syringomyeliques tardifs sus-lésionnels après traumatisme médullaire (à propos de trois observations cliniques). *Rev. Neurol.*, **106,** 751–755.

STERN, W. E. and RAND, R. W. (1959). Birth injuries to the spinal cord. *Amer. J. Obstet. Gynec.*, **78,** 498–512.

WAGNER, F. C., JR., DOHRMANN, G. J. and BUCY, P. C. (1971). Histopathology of transitory traumatic paraplegia in the monkey. *J. Neurosurg.*, **35,** 272–276.

WOLMAN, L. (1964). The neuropathology of traumatic paraplegia. A critical historical review. *Int. J. Paraplegia*, **1,** 233–251.

YASHON, D. and WHITE, R. J. (1974). Injuries of the vertebral column and spinal cord. In *Brock's Injuries of the Brain and Spinal Cord.* 5th edit. Ed. by E. H. Feiring. New York: Springer.

CHAPTER VI

INFLAMMATORY DISEASES

The protective encasement of the spinal cord within the meninges affords an important barrier to infective agents, but once these have gained access to the spinal cord, they encounter little resistance. The spinal fluid, lacking in cells and containing little immune protein, is an excellent culture medium for most organisms. For these reasons the situation of the infection, in relation to the various meningeal layers, is often as important as the type of organism concerned. This is particularly true of the common pyogenic bacteria which give rise, according to location, to intramedullary abscess, leptomeningitis, pachymeningitis, and extradural abscess. It might be thought that with the advent of antibiotics these types of pyogenic infections would be very rare. However the medical scene is continually changing and recently the prevalence of addiction to drugs taken by intramuscular or intravenous injection (Holzman and Bishko, 1971) has led to the appearance of a new important cause of septicaemia. Already spinal infections in drug addicts have been reported (Selby and Pillay, 1972). We shall deal separately with syphilis, tuberculosis and the rarer infections caused by fungi and parasites since these chronic infections have important differences from those caused by the acute pyogenic bacteria. In viral infections the situation is again different since these obligate intracellular parasites travel swiftly in their widespread involvement of tissue cells. They cause in the leptomeninges an acute meningitis which in many instances is of a benign nature. Within the spinal cord the attacks of certain viruses with a specific affinity for nerve cells give rise to some of the most serious diseases known in man.

BACTERIAL INFECTIONS

These include the clinicopathological states of extradural abscess, pachymeningitis, subdural abscess, leptomeningitis, and intramedullary abscess. In practice some of these conditions cannot be exactly distinguished and several may coexist. Leptomeningitis is by far the commonest and most important infection but, as coincidental and more serious involvement of the cerebral leptomeninges is the rule, this condition will only be dealt with briefly. A good review of non-specific leptomeningitis is that of Schleussing (1958).

Extradural (Epidural) Abscess

These abscesses may arise by direct extension from a neighbouring source of infection such as osteomyelitis of the spine, or by metastatic infection from an abscess elsewhere, or by the infection of a penetrating wound. Very occasionally no cause or source of infection can be found. Elsberg (1941) considered metastatic infection to be the commonest type. The clinical course commences with fever and pain in the back and progresses to paresis, sensory disturbance and bladder paralysis. The neurological involvement is usually due to pressure, and extension of the infection through the dura is unusual (Plum, 1962). The pathological finding is an abscess in the extradural space usually posteriorly situated and associated with osteomyelitis of the vertebral laminae. In the advanced cases the abscess behaves like a tumour and compresses the cord causing blockage of the subarachnoid space, and an increase of cells and protein in the spinal fluid. The changes induced in the spinal cord may be irreversible. The common organisms found in these abscesses have been *Staphylococcus aureus*, *Diplococcus pneumoniae*, and *Pseudomonas pyocyaneus*.

Pachymeningitis and Subdural Abscess

Some degree of pachymeningitis occurs in most cases of extradural abscess. It also occurs in conjunction with abscesses in the subdural space but these abscesses, also called intradural abscesses, are rare. They may occur following a penetrating wound, following a laminectomy operation, or may result from leptomeningitis with loculation of pus and rupture into the subdural space. Implantation of infection during the procedure of lumbar puncture has occasionally accounted for cases.

Pyogenic Leptomeningitis

The list of the types of bacteria which have been recorded as causing leptomeningitis is very large and Sahs and Joynt (1962) enumerate over twenty common organisms. There is a difference with age, for in adults *Neisseria meningitidis*, *Diplococcus pneumoniae*, *Streptococcus pyogenes*, and *Staphylococcus aureus* are the chief culprits whereas in infants and children the *Haemophilus influenzae* has been, in some series, the commonest pathogen.

Pseudomonas aeruginosa has now appeared as a common neurological pathogen due to contamination of intrathecal spinal punctures (Corbett and Rosenstern, 1971) or to hospital cross-infection (Ayliffe *et al.*, 1965). We shall deal here only with the pathological findings in the spinal cord.

The dura mater is usually normal. In the acute stage, the leptomeninges are opaque and filled out by a purulent exudate in the subarachnoid space. This exudate, of creamy-coloured pus, may be generalised or loculated but there is a tendency for it to be greatest on the posterior aspect, due probably to nursing of the patient in the supine position. In healed cases the leptomeninges remain opaque and these may be very thickened when the illness was protracted or inadequately treated with chemotherapy and antibiotics. The microscopical appearances are those expected in any purulent inflammation. There are many pus cells, polymorphs and bacteria. Lymphocytes and plasma cells are present in numbers dependent on the chronicity of the infection, which also determines the amount of fibroblasts and vascular connective tissue proliferation. The small vessels bathed in inflammatory exudate are affected by endarteritis and this may cause ischaemic damage to the spinal cord. Otherwise the spinal cord is unaffected unless there is grave infection with abscess formation.

Intramedullary Abscess

Intramedullary abscess of the spinal cord, whilst less common than its cerebral counterpart, had been recorded several times before the well-known case described by Chiari (1900). This was a man with bronchiectasis who developed metastatic spinal-cord abscesses together with cerebrospinal meningitis and a cerebellar abscess. Such cases are usually diagnosed at autopsy, but Woltman and Adson (1926) described recovery in an 11-year-old child following drainage of an encapsulated staphylococcal abscess of the thoracic cord. In a review of the literature they give descriptions of 29 similar cases of intramedullary abscesses. Betty and Lorber (1963) described two further cases and reviewed the intervening literature. Since this paper, the reports of Wright (1965), el Gindi and Fairburn (1969), Manfredi *et al.* (1970) and

Rifaat *et al.* (1973) have appeared. In most of the reported cases the intramedullary infection has been metastatic from a major source of pyogenic infection, e.g. bronchiectasis, although sometimes no apparent source has been discovered. A spinal abscess has followed a stab wound (Wright, 1965) and a high lumbar puncture (Rifaat *et al.*, 1973). These intramedullary abscesses of the spinal cord are often part of a syndrome of multiple septic foci. Leptomeningitis is frequently present and often there are coincident abscesses in the brain.

Intervertebral Disc Abscess

In addition to cases of osteomyelitis in which the inflammatory process involves the intervertebral disc there are occasional cases (Keiser and Grimes, 1963; Beattie, 1970; Rifaat *et al.*, 1973) in which there is an abscess more or less localised to the intervertebral disc. Some of these cases may present as a spinal osteomyelitis but others form a much more interesting group in that the clinical syndrome is that of a prolapsed intervertebral disc and often only histological and bacteriological studies reveal the infective nature of the disc pathology.

TUBERCULOSIS

The *Mycobacterium tuberculosis*, like the pyogenic bacteria, can affect different parts of the spinal canal and its contents. The two main conditions to be considered are the various manifestations of Pott's paraplegia and tuberculous leptomeningitis. For a full review of tuberculosis affecting the nervous system the reader is referred to Scheidegger (1958).

Pott's Paraplegia

Percivall Pott (1779) and David (1779) drew attention to the association of paraplegia with spinal curvature due to tuberculous caries. In Europe and North America serious paralysis from this cause is now rare and no longer presents a formidable problem to their orthopaedic services. But elsewhere and particularly in Asia, Africa and South America many cases remain untreated or inadequately treated. Griffiths *et al.* (1956) reviewed the morbid anatomical features of 86 cases in a full account of the clinical course and pathology of the condition. The mechanism by which the spinal cord is injured varies from case to case.

Extradural abscess.—The commonest state is a tuberculous osteitis of the vertebral bodies with an abscess in the extradural space causing compression of the spinal cord from its anterior aspect. The abscess may be composed of fluid pus, or of soft caseous material, or of firm tuberculous granulation tissue. The main effect on the spinal cord is that of pressure and the clinical course is rather similar to that caused by an extramedullary neoplasm except that clinical improvement may occur due to regression of the tuberculous process.

Bony disorders.—The bony disorders affect the spinal cord commonly in its thoracic portions (Fig. 41*a*, *b*). These range from a gradual angulation to a complete pathological dislocation and during this process a bony ridge or spur may form on the anterior wall of the spinal canal. Sequestra are formed from avascular portions of vertebral body or intervertebral disc and these add to the effect of the spur in narrowing the spinal canal. It must be emphasised that very considerable deformity of the canal can occur without paralysis which develops in these cases with bony disorder, because of the formation of bony spurs and sequestra.

Meningeal changes.—The dura mater often appears thickened but on closer examination what is usually found is a thick layer of tuberculous granulation tissue lying outside the intact and un-involved dura. In a series of 175 cases Griffiths *et al.* (1956) found no instance of interstitial tuberculous disease of the dura and concluded that in Pott's paraplegia tuberculous pachymeningitis is not an important factor in the causation of the paralysis. The tuberculous granulation tissue around the dura may contract and cause, by this cicatrising mechanism, constriction of the dural tube and its contents. This "peridural fibrosis" is an important surgical complication in Pott's disease; in the early cases the constriction of the cord can be relieved by stripping off the granulation tissue. Cases in which, following surgical correction of the deformed spinal canal, there is a relapse of the paraplegia, may have developed this "peridural fibrosis".

Spinal cord findings.—The commonest finding in the spinal cord in a case of Pott's paraplegia, unrelieved by surgical treatment, is a state of compression (Fig. 41*a*). There is deformity and in the compressed region loss of neurones and white matter. The lost cells and fibres are replaced by fibrous gliosis which outlines the area damaged by compression. The myelin loss is often gross and in the chronic cases with complete paraplegia there is often grotesque deformity of the spinal cord.

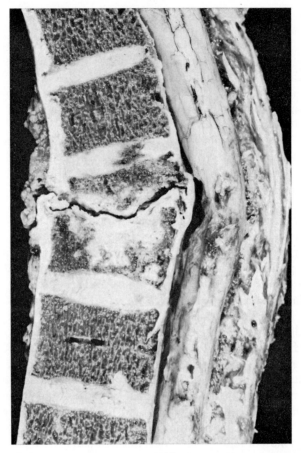

FIG. 41(*a*)

Spinal cord infarction.—One unusual but important complication of Pott's disease is infarction of the spinal cord. Seddon (1935) described a case of this and I have also made a necropsy on an example of this complication. The infarction arises by involvement of an important tributary vessel to the anterior spinal artery. The vessel concerned, which may be the vertebral or an intercostal or lumbar artery, is surrounded by the inflammatory reaction of a paravertebral abscess, which causes endarteritis and thrombosis.

Tuberculous Leptomeningitis

The advent of potent antituberculous drugs coupled with

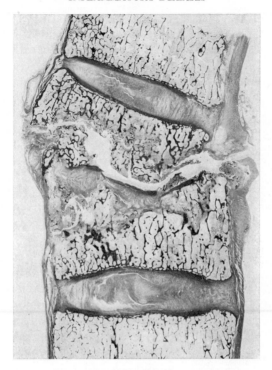

FIG. 41(b)

FIG. 41.—Pott's paraplegia. (a) Right half of a sagittally sawn specimen of thoracic cord. There is collapse of T7 and T8 vertebral bodies due to a tuberculous osteitis which has also spread into the T7–8 intervertebral disc. The anterior aspect of the spinal cord is compressed by the kyphosis. (b) Decalcified section of left half of spine seen in Fig. 41(a). The histological appearances are a mirror-image of Fig. 41(a).

energetic public health measures has dramatically diminished the incidence of this condition but it remains, nevertheless, a very important disease. The causative organism, *Mycobacterium tuberculosis* (usually of the human type), infects the leptomeninges (Rich and McCordock, 1933) by the rupture of an older tuberculous focus into the subarachnoid space. Experimentally the disease is reproduced readily by subarachnoid inoculation but not by intravenous administration of the bacilli. Often, at autopsy, the original focus cannot be found but sometimes one can observe a small caseous lesion in relation to the lateral ventricles of the cerebrum, the cortical meninges or the choroid plexus. Very rarely

(Sahs and Joynt, 1962) a small tuberculoma of the spinal cord is the primary focus in the nervous system.

Spinal cord findings.—The macroscopical appearance is that of a diffuse greyish opacity of the leptomeninges (Fig. 42). In a severe protracted case the whole spinal cord may be encircled with exudate (Fig. 43*a*, *b*). Small whitish 'tubercles' can usually be made out but often careful scrutiny is required. As in pyogenic leptomeningitis the exudate is more profuse on the posterior aspect of the cord. The spinal cord itself may be normal or softened depending on the degree of involvement of the small meningeal vessels.

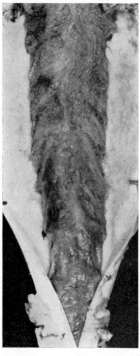

FIG. 42.—Posterior aspect of the upper cervical spinal cord of a case of tuberculous meningitis.

The microscopical appearance is that of a thick exudate in the subarachnoid space. In the majority of cases coming to necropsy (and which have survived several weeks) the exudate is at a stage where lymphocytes predominate. Poly-morphs are present in smaller numbers as are plasma cells. Epithelioid cells and multi-nucleated giant cells are always present but occur focally and sometimes require considerable search which, in my experience, has always revealed typical examples, although the bulk of the exudate may be lymphocytic. The finding of the tubercle bacilli usually is dependent on the amount of treatment given. In untreated cases they are always easy to find and may be very numerous indeed. But in cases having prolonged treatment, diagnostic acid-fast bacilli may be difficult or impossible to demonstrate. Culture and guinea-pig inoculation are much more reliable in diagnosis than histological staining for organisms, and should always be undertaken. Very rarely, and twice in the author's experience, one examines a spinal cord several years following successful treatment of a proven tuberculous leptomeningitis. The leptomeninges in these instances show only moderate opacity due to connective tissue thickening, and there is nothing to indicate the former disease process.

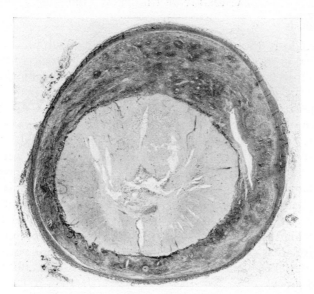

FIG. 43a.—Transverse section at T7 segmental level of the spinal cord of a case of tuberculous meningitis. Note the thick layer of exudate distending all the space within the dura and causing infarction of the spinal cord by endarteritis of the small spinal vessels. Haematoxylin and eosin × 5.

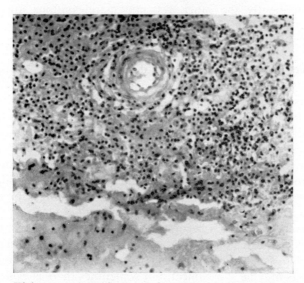

FIG. 43b.—High-power photomicrograph from the same slide as Fig. 43a, to show the endarteritis caused in small meningeal vessels buried in tuberculous exudate within the subarachnoid space. Haematoxylin and eosin × 160.

Sarcoidosis

Sarcoidosis (Scadding, 1967), a condition still presenting a problem in taxonomy, has such a common association with tuberculosis (among other diseases) that it is convenient to consider it here. It can affect the spinal cord in a similar manner to syphilis and tuberculosis. There are now many reports of sarcoidosis involving the central nervous system and among others those of Aszkanazy (1952), of Zeman (1958) and of Camp and Frierson (1962) illustrate the spinal cord involvement as seen at necropsy. The sarcoid lesions are granulomata composed of epithelioid cells, lymphocytes, giant cells, and occasionally plasma cells. These lesions are present in the leptomeninges around small meningeal vessels, and in the spinal cord itself again in relation to perivascular spaces (Fig. 44a, b). Related to the sarcoid granulomata are areas of localised spinal-cord necrosis due to ischaemia from arterial obliteration, or due to some other toxic effect of the sarcoid process.

Recently reports have appeared (Banerjee and Hunt, 1972; Semins et al., 1972) in which the clinical presentation is that of an expanding intramedullary tumour. Cases of sarcoidosis involving the nervous system can be difficult to diagnose the more so because frequently the other systemic manifestations are inconspicuous.

NEUROSYPHILIS

In recent years there has been a decline in cases of neurosyphilis not because syphilis itself has become uncommon, indeed recently there has been an alarming increase but because effective treatment originally by organic arsenicals and now by penicillin has usually contained the disease in its primary and secondary stage. The etiological agent (*Treponema pallidum*), first discovered in the primary lesion and its draining lymph nodes by Schaudinn and Hoffman (1905) and later found in the cerebrum of general paralysis cases by Noguchi and Moore (1913), is a motile spiral 5–20 microns long and 0.2 microns thick. Following infection, usually by sexual intercourse, it becomes rapidly disseminated throughout the body but invasion of the nervous system, an acute syphilitic meningitis, usually occurs in the so-called secondary stage. The meningitis may be sub-clinical, but sometimes there is evidence of meningeal irritation and there may be focal neurological signs. The spinal fluid shows a marked cellular increase with abnormal

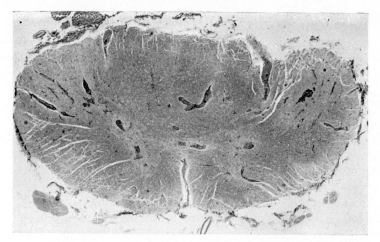

FIG. 44a.—Sarcoidosis. Transverse section through the thoracic part of the spinal cord of a case of sarcoidosis involving the central nervous system. Haematoxylin and Van Gieson ×11.

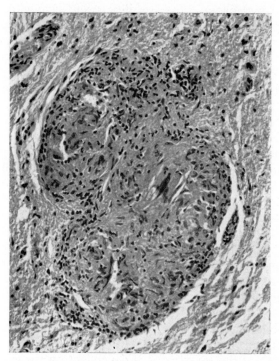

FIG. 44b.—High-power view of same case as in Fig. 44a. The picture shows an intramedullary granulomatous nodule of sarcoidosis. Haematoxylin and Van Gieson ×150.

globulins and a positive Wassermann reaction. In the rare necropsy cases examined in this stage (Pette, 1924) there is a diffuse meningitis with perivascular lymphocytic infiltration spreading into the spinal cord. Following this meningitic episode (which may be clinically silent) neurological involvement is considered to belong to the tertiary stage and is further sub-divided into meningovascular syphilis and parenchymal syphilis. In meningovascular syphilis there is a pronounced mesodermal reaction with a characteristic arteritis, the extent and situation of which largely determines the protean neurological damage. In parenchymal syphilis there is a direct effect on nervous tissue, possibly resulting from an altered tissue reaction to the spirochaete; this parenchymal form usually occurs later than meningovascular syphilis and by some authors is referred to as the quaternary stage of the disease. In the spinal cord, meningovascular syphilis gives rise to a variety of differing syndromes which I have grouped under the following headings: Syphilitic meningomyelitis, syphilitic pachymeningitis, syphilitic spastic paraplegia (Erb's), syphilitic amyotrophy. Parenchymal syphilis is represented in the spinal cord by tabes dorsalis.

Syphilitic Meningomyelitis (Fig. 45)

Excepting tabes dorsalis, the majority of cases of spinal syphilis fall into this category. The spinal cord is secondarily affected by involvement of the leptomeninges by a granulomatous exudate which, in its active phase, consists of microscopical gummata with central necrosis, macrophages with giant cells, and lymphocytes and plasma cells (Sträussler, 1958). A conspicuous feature is the arteritis that bears the name of Heubner (1874); although called an endarteritis obliterans it is really a panarteritis involving adventitia, media, and intima, probably in that sequence. Initially there is lymphocytic infiltration, later fibroblastic proliferation and finally collagenous thickening with narrowing of the lumen either concentrically or asymmetrically; at any of these stages a thrombosis may occur. This arterial lesion is often described as specific to syphilis but I do not agree there is any feature that is absent from arteritis due to other causes, e.g. tuberculous meningitis; in both the mechanism is the same, a reaction of the arterial wall to an inflammatory exudate.

The state of the spinal cord is dependent on the extent of the inflammatory exudate and the amount of arterial occlusion. The latter causes infarction with areas of necrosis of the spinal cord ranging in size from pinhead nodules of lipid phagocytes to large infarcted regions such as the territory of the anterior spinal artery. Although the lower thoracic and upper lumbar regions are most often involved, all parts of the cord can show lesions. A large laterally placed infarct will cause a hemitransection with a Brown–Séquard syndrome, whilst multiple scattered lesions result in a

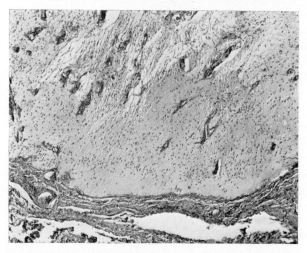

FIG. 45.—Meningovascular syphilis affecting the spinal cord. The picture shows a portion of the anterior white column seen in transverse section. Note the thickened leptomeninges and the necrosis with vascular proliferation in the spinal cord. Haematoxylin and eosin ×60.

well-recognised type called, from its macroscopical similarity to multiple sclerosis, syphilitic sclerosis. Another form caused by obliteration of small penetrating meningeal arteries has a concentric peripheral rim of infarction, the so-called syphilitic halo. The above picture refers to the active stage of inflammation and arterial obliteration; later the exudate is replaced by collagenous thickening of the leptomeninges and the spinal cord destruction proceeds to atrophy with areas of astrocytic gliosis.

Syphilitic Pachymeningitis

This is a form of hyperplastic gummatous meningitis first described by Charcot and Joffroy (1869) as pachymeningitis cervicalis hypertrophica. Despite the name, both pachymeninges and leptomeninges are involved in a granulomatous inflammation that welds the meningeal layers to the cord in a mass of fibrous granulation tissue. The cases of spinal block described by Froin (1903) were probably of this nature, for the clinical sequel is paraplegia with spinal root involvement and obliteration of the subarachnoid space. There are many clinical and pathological accounts of which those of Moniz (1925) and Gellerstedt (1956) may be recommended. The condition is moderately common but as cases frequently present unusual problems of diagnosis or treatment there is an annual appearance of case reports in the literature (Guidetti and La Torre, 1967; Wirth and Gado, 1973).

Erb's Syphilitic Spastic Paraplegia

This condition (Erb, 1892) is characterised clinically by a very slowly progressive paraparesis without sensory changes, the initial picture being that of gradually worsening bladder function. The pathology is thought to be discrete involvement of the fibres subserving bladder action; in the case of McMichael (1945) there was bilateral symmetrical degeneration of the posterolateral part of the lateral white columns seen in the lumbar and lower thoracic segments.

Syphilitic Amyotrophy

This name was given by the older neurologists to cases of syphilis mimicking motor neurone disease. The resemblance can be striking and both progressive muscular atrophy and amyotrophic lateral sclerosis can be simulated. Martin (1925) described the clincial features in sixty cases and the necropsy findings in two cases. As in other necropsy reports anterior horn atrophy was conspicuous but was combined with other features. The syphilitic halo of degeneration was marked in Martin's case 1. As a pathological entity syphilitic amyotrophy has less reality than as a clinical variant of neurosyphilis.

Tabes Dorsalis (Locomotor Ataxia)

No other spinal cord disorder has attracted such constant attention and controversy or bequeathed such a wealth of literature as tabes dorsalis. Even today when its clinical entity and relation to syphilis is proven many points of its pathogenesis remain disputed. The history of progress in understanding the disease is fascinating, but the references are so numerous (and often difficult of access) that for them the reader is referred to

Wilson (1954) and Gagel (1958); the latter account also contains the best recent description of the pathological findings.

From Hippocratic times the name tabes signified some wasting disease, but by the nineteenth century it was clear from the writings of Hutin, Cruveilhier and Ollivier that the term had taken the meaning of a spinal ataxia. In the eighteen-fifties the pathological finding of posterior column gliosis was referred to by Todd,

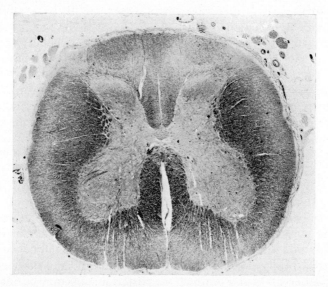

FIG. 46.—Tabes dorsalis. Transverse section, stained for myelin, at L5 segmental level, of a spinal cord from an early case of tabes dorsalis. Note the pattern of the posterior column degeneration and the rim of myelin pallor in the anterior and lateral white columns. Weil × 13.

Romberg, Turck and Rokitansky; then followed a spate of papers claiming or denying the syphilitic etiology of tabes dorsalis. This question was resolved correctly by Gowers in England, Fournier in France and Erb in Germany, but proof was lacking until the demonstration of the spirochaete by Noguchi. For a full clinical account the reader is referred to Wilson (1954); here I shall only mention the ataxia, lightning pains, pupillary changes and loss of deep tendon reflexes.

Pathological findings in tabes dorsalis (Fig. 46).—Significant changes are most evident in the spinal cord and meninges; they occur regularly in the posterior nerve roots, but have only occasionally been reported in the posterior root ganglia. The leptomeninges are affected by fibrous thickening which is significantly greater posteriorly. This is accompanied by a variable amount of lymphocytic and plasma cell infiltration; such changes in relation to the root sleeves will be discussed later. In a severe case of tabes the grey gliosis of the posterior columns is striking and the accompanying atrophy may visibly alter the shape of the spinal cord. In an early or mild case, fibres subserving the lower thoracic and lumbosacral regions are chiefly affected though these upwardly degenerating fibres will be seen in all segments cephalad.

Pierret in 1871 (quoted by Greenfield, 1963) considered the pattern of fibre degeneration in these cases distinctive and following the embryological work of Flechsig (1876) it was considered that these early myelinating fibres were axons from cell bodies in Clarke's column, and that tabes was a system degeneration involving these fibres. This question has never been resolved; personally I have observed very similar fibre degeneration patterns in tabes and in cases of posterior rhizotomy, and I find it unnecessary to postulate damage to wholly intraspinal nerve fibres. The posterior nerve roots are commonly reported to show atrophy with depletion of nerve fibres; in my experience this is a constant finding but some early reports deny root involvement. Of course Wallerian degeneration of posterior column fibres will be associated with atrophy of posterior roots which are caudal to the segment under observation and of which the posterior roots may be normal; this may account for the few discrepant reports. Minor changes in the posterior root ganglia have been described usually as shrinkage or depletion of neurones rather than inflammation. A few reports mention degeneration in peripheral nerves and in the autonomic nervous system.

Theories of pathogenesis.—Two problems confront us, the nature of the syphilitic effect and the site of its action. With regard to the former, opinion is now against regarding the disease as a system degeneration, preferring to regard the nerve degeneration as secondary to damage by syphilitic granulation tissue. Three sites for the point of fibre damage have been suggested.

(i) *Intraspinal.*—This was in the earlier accounts the most popular theory but it has not withstood the abundant later reports of posterior root atrophy, a change not expected from a spinal lesion.

(ii) *Intraganglionic.*—The objection to this site, championed by Marinesco and Oppenheim, is that the changes found in the posterior root ganglion are minor and probably secondary to axon interruption elsewhere.

(iii) *Posterior nerve root.*—This remains the likeliest site but even here two locations on the root are suggested. Obersteiner and Redlick in 1894 (quoted by Wilson, 1954) put the lesion at the entry of the posterior root into the spinal cord. Here the fibres lose their neurilemmal sheath and it is thought are more vulnerable to syphilitic attack. The alternate location on the root was put forward by Nageotte (1903) who found significant changes, later confirmed by Richter and by Hechst (1931), on the portion of posterior nerve root between the end of the pia-arachnoid sleeve and the ganglion. This portion of the root is called the radicular nerve of Nageotte. The changes were those of syphilitic granulation tissue in which Pick found spirochaetes.

FUNGAL INFECTIONS

Several types of fungi may involve the spinal cord either as a complication of a debilitating, possibly malignant, disease or as a primary infection of the central nervous system. Although rare these diseases are extremely serious and until recently were usually fatal. Torulosis is the commonest reported condition but coccidioidomycosis, histoplasmosis, blastomycosis and aspergillosis account for a few cases.

For a general review of fungal infections the reader is referred to the work edited by Wolstenholme and Porter (1968).

Torulosis (Cryptococcosis)

The etiological agent (*Cryptococcus hominis*) is a spherical or oval yeast-like organism whose size is usually in the range 4–7 microns (Littman and Zimmerman, 1956). This fungus is widespread in nature throughout the world and causes a mycotic infection of man and animals due to airborne carriage into the respiratory passages from a reservoir in the soil. From the lungs it appears to be disseminated in the blood stream to all parts of the body including the central nervous system, which is particularly susceptible to the infection. The commonest form is a granulomatous leptomeningitis and, although the spinal meninges are concomitantly affected, the cerebral state is the more important.

The diagnosis during life is usually made by the recognition of the organisms in the CSF. Unless budding forms can be seen, crypto-cocci can be mistaken for lymphocytes and a technique using Indian ink to show the morphology in relief is useful. If the orga-nisms are scanty they can be concentrated by filtration of CSF through a millipore and they can also be cultured. Cryptococcal antigen can be detected in the CSF by complement fixation techniques and by a latex agglutination test (Goodman et al., 1971). For a description and review of cryptococcal leptomen-ingitis and cerebral granulomata the reader is referred to Matheis (1960). Here we shall mention only the reports with predominant involvement of the spinal cord. These cases have a large granulo-matous mass which may be situated outside or inside the dura or may be intramedullary.

In the cases of Smith and Crawford (1930), Fitchett and Weid-man (1934), Reeves et al. (1941), and Matheis (1960), involvement of the spinal cord or the cauda equina was demonstrated at autopsy. The usual finding was a large necrotic mass that could be in the extradural space, in the centre of the cord or intradurally among the nerve roots of the cauda equina. Cases explored surgically and having a similar variety of lesions were reported by Carton and Mount (1951), Ley et al. (1951), Alajouanine et al. (1953), Ramamurthi and Anguli (1954), and Skultety (1961). Frequently leptomeningitis coexists or follows the development of the localised granuloma. Histologically the lesions are those of an inflammatory granuloma with multinucleated giant cells. There is no true casea-tion but necrosis does occur and a gelatinous exudate is common. The inflammatory cells are chiefly lymphocytes with a few plasma cells. The organisms are encapsulated yeast-like forms either free or within macrophages. In most cases the cryptococci are present in very large numbers and their demonstration is easy. In cases of diagnostic difficulty some of the procedures described earlier might be tried.

Histoplasmosis

Histoplasmosis, caused by *Histoplasma capsulatum*, is a mycotic infection involving the reticulo-endothelial system of various organs and tissues. Geographically, the disease has a widespread distribution, and is endemic in the Mississippi and Ohio valleys, with many other areas in the United States of epidemic and sporadic occurrence. Cases have been reported in Central and South America, Europe, Africa, Asia, and Australia. The organism, in the regions concerned, infects soil and is known to be excreted in the droppings of pigeons, starlings and bats. The entry of the organism in human cases is by inhalation and in a susceptible person there is a lesion in the lungs and the hilar lymph nodes, rather similar to the primary complex of tuberculosis. In the United States, histoplasmosis is a common infection occurring yearly in tens of thousands of new cases (Schwarz and Baum, 1963). The majority of infections are trivial and may be asymptomatic, but in some cases there is progressive disseminated infection of serious degree. Only rarely is the central nervous system involved and Schulz (1953) in a review of 120 reported cases with necropsy found mention of such involvement in only twelve cases. Shapiro et al. (1955) reviewing their own necropsy material found lesions in brain or meninges in six out of eleven cases of histoplasmosis. Juba (1958) and Nelson et al. (1961) have reported two further instances, and, in the case of the latter authors, recovery followed the use of the drug amphotericin B.

The pathological findings are those of a chronic granulomatous leptomeningitis with small granulomata situated in relation to small veins. Occasionally a large "histoplasmoma" has been reported in the brain but only with disseminated infections. I know of no case in which the disease was predominantly affecting the spinal cord. The organisms are round or oval, single or budding spores measuring 1 to 3 microns in diameter, Gram-positive and acid-fast in their staining. Some are free but many are in macrophages either unattached or surrounding small vessels.

Coccidioidomycosis

The etiological agent of this disease, *Coccidioides immitis*, is a hardly filamentous fungus which thrives in the soil of relatively arid regions in California, New Mexico, Arizona, Texas, Nevada, Utah and in the northern states of Mexico (Littman et al., 1958). The organism is known to cause disease in sheep, cattle, dogs, and various wild rodents. In residents or even travellers in these regions the disease is very common. A recent epidemic (Werner et al., 1972) affected 61 out of 103 archeology students excavating Indian ruins near Chico in California. The usual course of the disease is a mild febrile infection. Rarely (Bruschi, 1961) there is a serious progressive disease to which Negroes and Filipinos are more prone than are Caucasians.

There are many reports of involvement of the brain and spinal cord, which may be affected by a granulomatous leptomeningitis with or without small granulomata in the nervous parenchyma. The spinal cord may also be involved by extradural granulomata developing from infective foci in the spine. Cases of this nature were described by Rand (1930) and by Jackson *et al.* (1964). The histological lesions, of giant-celled granulomata, are not very different from those of other fungi or of tuberculosis. The organism, in tissues, is found in macrophages or in the large giant cells as large thick-walled spherules 10–80 microns in diameter and made up of many endospores 2–5 microns in diameter.

Blastomycosis

North American blastomycosis is caused by *Blastomyces dermatidis*, whilst in South America a similar infection is caused by *Blastomyces brasiliensis*. *Blastomyces dermatidis* (Schwarz and Baum, 1951) is a double-walled, single-budding yeast cell 5–20 microns in size, growing as a yeast at 37°C, but as a mycelium at room temperature. Blastomycosis is a chronic granulomatous infection commonly involving the skin and subcutaneous tissues. The reservoir of infection is soil and the disease mainly affects male workers engaged in agriculture. The disease occasionally involves the lungs and more rarely spreads by the blood stream to involve other viscera, bone, and the central nervous system. The brain and spinal cord may be involved directly or there may be an acute or chronic leptomeningitis often with a course similar to tuberculosis meningitis. Involvement of the spinal cord was mentioned by Solway *et al.* (1939), Craig *et al.* (1940), and by Greenwood and Voris (1950).

The case reported by Osmond *et al.* (1971) presented to an orthopaedic centre as a case of osteomyelitis of the spine causing paraplegia. The authors were familiar with this mode of presentation from other cases occurring in their part of Africa (Durban).

The spinal cord may be involved in a generalised leptomeningitis, but more often a case with paraplegia has a blastomycotic abscess of a vertebra and involving the spinal canal. In such cases the spinal cord is damaged by pressure as well as by direct inflammation. The microscopical picture is a mixture of acute and chronic inflammation and in this respect differs from tuberculosis. Other features such as the areas of necrosis and the many multinucleated giant cells are very similar to tuberculosis. Fortunately for diagnosis, the causative organisms are usually prominent. They may be free or within large phagocytes and their structure is that of yeasts which divide by single-budding division only. The organism has a double contour but this is not a capsule stainable by toluidine blue as in the morphologically similar cryptococcus.

Aspergillosis

Disease caused by the fungus *Aspergillus fumigatus* is uncommon but the incidence is increasing because of the modern iatrogenic causes of diminished host resistance to normally saprophytic fungi. In fresh smear preparations and on histological examination the organism appears as a mycelium with distinctive conidiophore structures identifiable by an expert mycologist. Culture is also possible but one difficulty in interpretation is the ubiquity of contaminating spores of similar fungal forms.

There are many reports of involvement of the central nervous system by *Aspergillus fumigatus* and the list which follows is a selection: Iyer *et al.* (1952), Jackson *et al.* (1955), Burston and Blackwood (1963), Hughes (1966), Mukoyama *et al.* (1969) and Seres *et al.* (1972).

There is a range of clinical presentation of the cases both of the variety of the fungal infection and also of the clinical setting which often involves a background disease and its treatment. There may be a chronic granulomatous meningitis or meningo-encephalitis, or the brain or spinal cord may be the seat of solitary or multiple granulomata. Some cases (Mukoyama *et al.* (1969) have a large brain abscess.

The spinal cord is frequently involved in the infection and sometimes is predominantly affected. In the case of Seres *et al.* (1972) aspergillosis caused an inflammatory mass of the thoracic spine and this led to compression of the spinal cord.

PARASITIC INFESTATIONS

The main parasitic conditions which give rise to a localised involvement of the spinal cord are cysticercosis, hydatid disease and schistosomiasis. In certain areas of the world paragonimiasis and gnathostomiasis cause dramatic spinal cord syndromes. In many other parasitic diseases the spinal cord is affected but only as part of a general infestation of the central nervous system, and for a detailed account of these and other rare infective agents the following references are suggested: *Trichiniasis*, Fischer (1955) and Escobar and Nieto (1972); *Malaria*, Scheidegger (1958a); *Toxoplasmosis*, Scheidegger (1958b) and Frenkel (1972); and *Trypanosomiasis*, van Bogaert (1958) and Manuelidis (1972).

Cysticercosis

This disease results from the ingestion by man of the ova of the pork tapeworm, *Taenia solium*. The emerging embryos penetrate the intestinal wall and become widely disseminated throughout the body. They may live for a few years, but then die and become calcified. The human disease, cysticercosis, is a variant in the life cycle for otherwise the embryos, developing in the pig, are eaten by man who then harbours the adult stage in his intestine—taeniasis. Cysticercosis is particularly prevalent where the pig is a favourite food and in regions where hygiene is primitive. The disease is common in Poland and Germany, and large series of cases have been observed in Mexico, South America, and India. Cysticercosis affects the central nervous system in two ways. The dissemination of the embryos often results in cysts in the brain and occasionally in the spinal cord, and in these locations they grow, then die and calcify. In the brain these cysts give rise to epileptic attacks, whilst in the spinal cord they cause focal lesions. The other type of cysticercosis is called the racemose form and in this there are multiple cysts grouped together like grapes. This type of infestation is seen in the cerebral ventricles and in the subarachnoid space and, when occurring at the base of the brain, causes hydrocephalus. Similar examples may occur in the spinal subarachnoid space. Reports of spinal cord cysticercosis are few and it is probable that a thorough search in this situation is rarely made. Fischer (1955) refers to three cases known to him and specific spinal cord localisation was seen in the cases reported by Rosenblath (1913), Dazzi and Verga (1926) Korbsch (1932), and Hesketh (1965). The case reported by Kahn (1972) was unusual in that a syndrome of amyotrophic lateral sclerosis was present.

The pathological findings differ in the two types of the disease. In the first type there are round, thick-walled, cysts in the subdural space, the subarachnoid space or within the cord (Fig. 47*a*, *b*). Their histological structure depends on the period that has elapsed since the death of the embryo. The cyst of a live embryo evokes only

---

FIG. 47.—Cysticercosis of the spinal cord. Case of Hesketh (1965). (*a*) Photomicrograph of cyst excised from the spinal cord, ×35. (*b*) Enlargement of part of parasite seen in Fig. 47*a*. The picture shows the scolex, ×160.

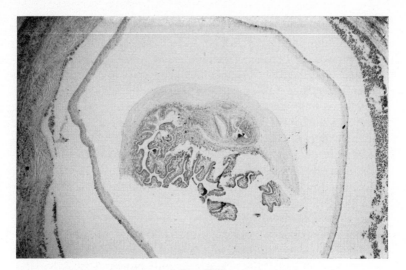

FIG. 47(a)

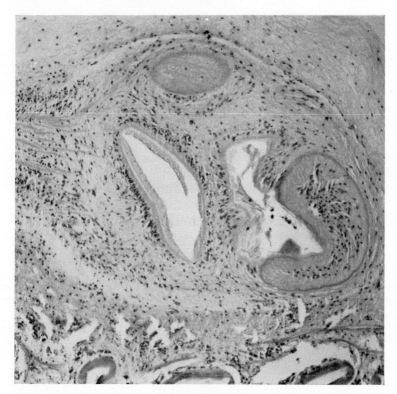

FIG. 47(b)

a slightly inflammatory reaction and gliosis. After death the cyst is surrounded by a zone of polymorphs, lymphocytes and multinucleated giant cells. A zone of fibrous tissue forms and this eventually heals as a thick collagenous capsule, which may calcify. The embryo has usually died and has been absorbed at the stage these cases are observed. In the racemose form the embryos are frequently alive and have the form of small clear, glistening, ovoid bladders about 0.5 cm in diameter. At one side there is invagination within which is the head with its diagnostic hooklets.

Hydatid Disease

This disease is caused by the larval form of the parasite *Taenia echinococcus*, whose life cycle is concerned with the sheep and the dog. The disease is rare in Great Britain and in the United States but common in Australia, New Zealand, North Africa, Iceland, Uruguay and Argentina. The adult cestode lives in the intestine of the dog and human infection results from ingestion of the ova which are excreted in very large numbers in the dog faeces. The embryos, which hatch in the stomach and intestines, burrow through the gut wall and enter the portal venous system by which they reach the liver. They may pass through the liver and lungs, becoming widely disseminated throughout the body and forming what are called primary hydatid cysts. The liver is the commonest organ involved and from the developed primary cysts, in the liver or elsewhere, secondary or metastatic hydatic cysts may arise when the original mature cysts rupture and liberate the contained daughter cysts. The central nervous system may be involved in both types of the disease, but the majority of cases are metastatic from liver or lung infection. The spinal cord is involved either by a direct primary or metastatic cyst, or more commonly by vertebral involvement and pressure effects due to extension into the spinal canal. Fischer (1955) estimated that about a dozen cases of cysts within the spinal cord had been reported, whilst there were at least 200 reports of involvement of the vertebrae and spinal canal. Reports dealing specifically with spinal cord involvement have been published by Brütt (1931), Popov and Umerow (1935), Cosacesco and Vereano (1946), and Hesketh (1965).

The size of the cysts is 2 to 10 cm according to age and situation. The cyst wall is made up by a chitinous substance forming a laminated ectocyst of considerable thickness and giving the characteristic grey appearance. Within this is an inner membrane, the germinative membrane, which is seen only microscopically. Within this are brood capsules containing scolices measuring about 150 μm in diameter. The scolices have minute invaginated heads with rows of hooklets. The nature of these cysts can often be ascertained by microscopy of the aspirated fluid and seeing the hooklets in the fine sediment called hydatid sand. Surrounding the cysts is a dense connective tissue and chronic inflammatory layer, and when the cyst is intramedullary this has a surrounding glial reaction.

Schistosomiasis

This disease is caused by infestation by any of three members of a group of trematode parasites. Man is the primary host and the secondary host is a water snail whose species differs for each trematode. The three parasites that commonly give rise to human diseases are *Schistosoma haematobium*, found mainly in Africa; *S. mansoni*, found in Africa but also in South America; and *S. japonicum*, found in the Far East. In the case of *S. japonicum*, cattle, horse, goat, dog and cat can be the primary host and suffer the same disease as man. The life cycle of these parasites is complex. The ovum, excreted in urine or faeces of human cases, in water becomes a swimming miracidium which enters the secondary host, the water snail. In this host the bifid-tailed cercariae are produced, which can enter the human skin during washing or bathing or may be ingested in drinking water. Following invasion of the human primary host the adult worms are formed in the liver and then migrate to the bladder (*S. haematobium*), rectum (*S. mansoni*), or mesenteric, colonic and rectal veins (*S. japonicum*). Involvement of the central nervous system is rare and there are interesting differences between the various types of parasites. *Schistosoma haemotobium* predominantly affects the spinal cord, *S. mansoni* causes lesions equally either in the brain or in the spinal cord, whilst *S. japonicum* affects (with 2 reported exceptions) only the brain. It is not known why this striking species difference is maintained in the relative involvement of brain and spinal cord. Wakefield *et al.* (1962) considered that the gravid female schistosome migrated from the pelvic veins to the vertebral veins via the anastomatic venous system demonstrated by Batson (1940).

Cases of spinal cord involvement by schistosomiasis have been reported by Müller and Stender (1930), Day and Kenawy (1936), Hoff and Shaby (1939), Gama and de Sa (1945), Faust (1948) Ross *et al.* (1952), Maciel *et al.* (1954), Pepler and Lombaard

(1958), Hutton and Holland (1960), Wakefield *et al.* (1962), Budzilovich *et al.* (1964), Bird (1964), Odeku *et al.* (1968), Sennara (1969) and Herskowitz (1972).

According to Herskowitz the world literature contains 104 cases of schistosomiasis of the central nervous system. Of the 30 cases due to *S. mansoni* 11 involved only the brain and 19 only the spinal cord. Of the 14 cases caused by *S. haematobium* 3 involved the brain, 9 the spinal cord and 2 involved both brain and cord.

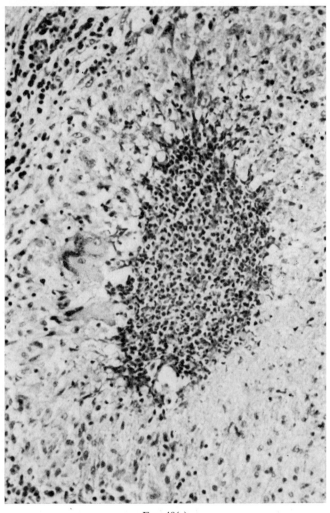

Fig. 48(*a*)

Schistosoma japonicum has caused 60 reported cases of which 58 affected only the brain, 1 only the cord and 1 both the brain and cord.

The most common levels of spinal cord involvement are the low thoracic region, the lumbar enlargement and less often the cauda equina. The parasitic infestation of the theca may cause a radiculopathy or a myelopathy.

The clinical syndrome begins with pains in the back and legs and in the space of two or three weeks paraparesis develops and progresses to paraplegia with appropriate loss of sensation and paralysis of bowel and bladder. Eosinophilia of the blood is common and eosinophils may occur in the cerebrospinal fluid.

The necropsy reports do not include any description of a walled-off parasitic cyst. Instead they refer to softened areas of the lumbosacral enlargement (Fig. 48a and b). The histological findings are

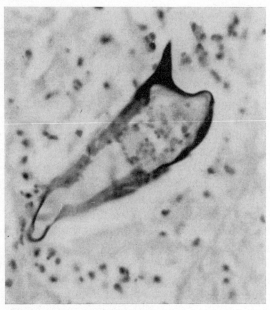

FIG. 48(*b*)

FIG. 48.—Schistosomiasis of the spinal cord. Case of Herskowitz (1972). (*a*) Low-power photomicrograph of granulomatous lesion in the conus medullaris. The centre of the lesion contains polymorphs and necrotic debris. The intermediate zone is composed of many epithelioid cells and a few multinucleated cells of Langhans type. Haematoxylin and eosin ×8.

(*b*) Photomicrograph of a Schistosoma egg within the conus medullaris. Note the lateral spine identifying the Mansoni type.

those of an acute necrotic haemorrhagic myelitis. Much (
tissue destruction is due to infarction both venous and ar
Ova can be seen within small intramedullary veins whic
undergoing thrombophlebitis. The arterioles are also af
(Maciel *et al.*, 1954) with necrotic fibrinoid degeneration le
to oedema and haemorrhage. These changes are attributed
toxic effect of the ova and this toxicity is exerted also di
against the nervous tissue of the spinal cord. The response
host may vary since in Case 1 of Budzilovich *et al.* (196
reaction was observed around the ova. The ova of these par
are diagnostic; that of *S. haematobium* is oval, measures 140
microns and has a short terminal spine at one end; the c
S. mansoni are oval, rather larger and with a single lateral
(Fig. 48*b*). The ovum of *S. japonicum* is oval, measures 80 ×
and has a small rudimentary spine or knob near one end.

Paragonimiasis

The disease paragonimiasis is caused by a lung fluke
genus Paragonimus and occurs in Asia, Africa and South Am
The disease is endemic in Korea, Japan and China, and
pathological studies of the disease affecting the brain and
cord (Oh, 1968 and 1969) have been made on cases in k
Paragonimus westermani is the prevalent species in Asia
mature fluke of *P. westermani* is oval and measures 7.5–1
by 4–6 mm. It is covered by spiny processes and has two su
The eggs are pear-shaped and measure approximately 100 ×

The human disease is caused by infestation by the adult
The life cycle of the parasite involves a species of snail an
various crustacea. Human infection arises from eating r
imperfectly cooked crab or crayfish. The ingested cer
penetrate the intestinal wall and probably enter the pleural
from the peritoneal cavity by burrowing through the diaph
They enter the lungs which are the main site of infestation.
sites are the brain (30–60 per cent), spinal cord and v
subcutaneous regions. Cerebral paragonimiasis is comm
Korea where it accounts for almost a quarter of space-occu
intracerebral lesions.

Spinal paragonimiasis is uncommon even in endemic ar
pulmonary paragonimiasis. According to Oh (1969) about 4
of spinal paragonimiasis have been reported. These cases p

with a progressive paraparesis which may take weeks or months to become a complete cord transection. The lower thoracic region is that commonly affected and the presentation is that of a spastic paraplegia with sensory loss below the appropriate segmental level. More rarely the lesion is in the lumbosacral enlargement, causing a flaccid paraplegia. Occasionally there is involvement of the cauda equina and sometimes the presenting signs suggest the diagnosis of a herniated disc. In the common lower thoracic cases there is usually a spinal block demonstrable by manometric testing and by myelography.

The presentation of a case with the features just described at a surgical or neurosurgical centre usually leads to a laminectomy. The disease is seen either as a granulomatous mass or as spreading inflammatory tissue in the epidural space. The abnormal tissue can often be evacuated with a relatively good prognosis. The histological appearance of the excised tissue is that of chronic inflammatory granulation tissue often with calcification and with a lymphocyte and plasma cell reaction. The diagnosis depends on the finding and the recognition in the tissue of the adult fluke or of the ova. There are many morphological features (Sawitz, 1956) distinguishing this fluke from *Fasciola hepatica*. Distinguishing the ova of *P. westermani* from those of *F. hepatica* and *S. japonicum* is more difficult but there are (Faust and Russel, 1957) distinguishing features.

Gnathostomiasis

A type of eosinophilic myeloencephalitis prevalent in Thailand has been shown to be caused by the burrowing activities in and around the brain and spinal cord of the adult form of a nematode called *Gnathostoma spinigerum* (Bunnag *et al.*, 1970). This worm infests the stomach wall of dogs and cats, and man is infected by eating raw or imperfectly cooked small animals such as frogs, fish and chickens, which harbour the larvae.

The clinical course of the neurological disease is dramatic, beginning with severe pain over the trunk or limbs which in a few days gives way to paralysis or sensory loss. The blood picture shows an eosinophilia. The necropsy examination of the brain and spinal cord shows many large necrotic and haemorrhagic tracks of the burrowing organism. Subarachnoid, intracerebral and intraventricular haemorrhages are common.

VIRUS DISEASES
We are concerned here chiefly with the neurotropic viruses, a category in which are grouped those viruses with a particular affinity for nerve cells. This affinity is not an immutable characteristic and these diseases may involve other tissues, e.g. the salivary adenitis of rabies. Also in different species the behaviour of the same virus may change and its neurotropism may be either more or less displayed. Following laboratory "passage" a certain strain of virus may change, in its neurotropic properties, for a certain species. A large number of viruses have been shown to involve or been suspected of involving the spinal cord or its meninges, but in only a few of these is the spinal-cord involvement a prominent feature. Of these I have selected for detailed description the viruses of rabies, anterior poliomyelitis, herpes zoster and herpes-B encephalomyelitis. Kuru and Jakob-Creutzfeldt disease are also included as examples of 'slow virus diseases', a recently recognised form of transmissible but slowly developing degenerative disease of the nervous system (Whitty et al., 1969). For a more general account of virus infections of the central nervous system the reader is referred to the reviews of Bieling and Poetschke (1958) and of Nieberg and Blumberg (1972).

Rabies (Hydrophobia, Lyssa, La Rage, Tollwut)
This is an endemic disease of carnivores which, having a salivary gland infection, transmit the disease by biting. The possible reservoir of infection includes dogs, wolves, foxes, coyotes, skunks, vampire bats and several other smaller vectors. Most mammals can contract the disease and in man a fatal encephalomyelitis ensues. The human disease is prevalent in eastern Europe, Asia, Africa, locally in parts of North and South America, and (Lassen, 1962) in Greenland. It is now spreading westwards through Europe with occasional large outbreaks as in Amsterdam (Noordam, 1963). Great Britain had almost eradicated the disease by her quarantine of imported dogs, introduced in 1897, but is now again threatened by rabies. Since 1918 there have been 5 confirmed cases of human rabies in Britain but all have arisen by infection contracted before arrival from abroad. For a recent review of the world distribution of animal and human rabies the monograph of Bisseru (1972) should be consulted.

Etiological agent.—Galloway and Elford (1936) estimated by a filtration technique the size of the rabies virus to be 100–150 nm.

As shown experimentally by Pasteur, following the bite, it travels neurotropically along peripheral nerve trunks, and eventually (in days or months) can be demonstrated throughout the central and peripheral nervous system as well as in salivary glands and often in other organs. It has been found in adrenals, spleen, kidney, liver, lung, testicle, myocardium, pancreas and eye. The virus can be recovered from saliva, urine, milk and blood.

Negri bodies.—These structures, specific to rabies and originally demonstrated by Negri (1903), are intracytoplasmic bodies seen in neurones, the most constant being the pyramidal cells of the hippocampus. In a suspected animal the hippocampus should be examined by the fresh impression method of Sellers (1927). The bodies measure from 5–10 μm, and they are well-defined, round eosinophilic structures containing basophilic granules. Eosinophilic bodies without basophilic granules are called Lyssa bodies; they may have the same significance but unlike Negri bodies they are not specific to rabies. Negri bodies may also be found in the neurones of the cerebral cortex, basal ganglia, cranial nerve nuclei, spinal cord, posterior root ganglia and the ganglia of the sympathetic nervous system. They are often absent from many of these sites particularly after laboratory passage.

General necropsy findings.—Terminal changes may obscure the picture but in many organs there is hyperaemia, and inflammatory changes have been described, particularly in the salivary glands from which virus has been recovered (Berntsen and Stevenson, 1953). The appearances in the brain were described by Schükri and Spatz (1925), and the large literature reviewed by Sükrü-Aksel (1958). The encephalitis is related in severity to the rapidity of the clinical course. Particularly affected are the substantia nigra, the nuclei around the third and fourth ventricles and the aqueduct, but the jugular and Gasserian ganglia are also involved. The damaged nerve cells show changes ranging from chromatolysis to neuronophagia with clusters of polymorphs and microglia around the dead neurones forming the aggregates known as Babés bodies.

Findings in the spinal cord.—In the paralytic form of rabies, the spinal cord changes predominate. There is evidence that the part of the cord affected is related to the site of inoculation and certainly in the Trinidad cases of Hurst and Pawan (1931 and 1932), when the victims were bitten in the feet by vampire bats, the spinal cord was mainly involved. The spinal cord is congested and soft. Microscopically an intense myelitis is present with morphs, lymphocytes and microglial cells. In the grey n both anterior and posterior horns are equally affected, neurones showing chromatolysis or dissolution from neu phagia with a marked microglial proliferation spreading in white matter. In the peripheral white matter small foci of mic are present and in the Virchow-Robin spaces an exuda lymphocytes and polymorphs is present not however spre to any extent into the leptomeninges. In none of the ca Hurst and Pawan were Negri bodies demonstrable. The diag can now be confirmed by fluorescent antibody techniques (wasser and Kissling, 1958).

Acute Anterior Poliomyelitis (Heine-Medin Disease, Inf Paralysis, Kinderlähmung, Poliomyélite)

In the Carlsberg Glyptothek at Copenhagen is a limeston of the XVIIIth Dynasty (2000 B.C.) which depicts the priest who has an atrophied leg suggestive of childhood anterior myelitis. The disease was probably known to Hippocrat there is a reference in his writings to epidemic paraplegia.

The first account in the later European medical literat thought to be that of Underwood (1789); there are several vening accounts (Paul, 1829; Badham, 1834) but that of (1840) is noteworthy for his excellent clinical account c disease. The first important description of the pathological fin in the spinal cord was that of Charcot and Joffroy (1870) w their case accurately correlated the pattern of muscular at with the neuronal loss in the spinal cord. There have been later accounts of the spinal cord pathology, but notew were those of Wickman (1913) who studied five cases and Ho Hechst's (1935) description of 28 cases. For a review c literature and a detailed account of the spinal cord chang reader is referred to Baker and Cornwell (1956), Van B (1958) and Bodian (1959).

Etiological agent.—Landsteiner and Popper (1909) estab the responsible agent as a virus, its size being estimated by I et al. (1935) as 8–12 nm though electron microscopy gives s larger values. Three strains are recognised, now called I, II and III (Bodian et al., 1949), but formerly termed Bru (after a chimpanzee), Lansing (after a Michigan town), and (after a Californian patient). Type I is the most common, T gives rise to milder attacks but is pathogenic to rats, mice and hamsters. Types I and III are only pathogenic to primates but will grow in tissue cultures of monkey or human tissues.

Epidemiology and clinical course.—Poliomyelitis is a widespread endemic and epidemic disease mainly of white races in temperate climates (white races are also highly susceptible in the tropics) and occurring naturally only in human populations. The disease is contracted by ingestion of food or water contaminated by infected faeces, either directly from human subclinical cases or from sewage effluents or carried by house or blow flies. Clinical involvement of the nervous system occurs only in a small proportion of cases harbouring the virus who otherwise experience only a mild alimentary tract infection with regional lymph node involvement but no viraemia (Bodian, 1959). Viraemia and invasion of the central nervous system occurs in a small proportion of cases and trauma (e.g. tonsillectomy, subcutaneous injections) or excessive exercise may act by localising the site of nervous system involvement. The route by which the nervous system is invaded is not known, although in animal experiments spread along nerve trunks can be demonstrated. The spinal fluid changes vary with the stage of the disease; initially there are up to 200 cells per mm^3 of which 50 per cent may be polymorphs, and the protein is slightly raised. When the paralytic stage ensues (approximately two weeks after infection) the cell count drops to 10–20 lymphocytes per mm^3 whilst the protein steadily rises up to 200 mg/100 ml and may remain at a high level for many months.

General necropsy findings.—Terminal changes are often present but the only specific pathology described outside the nervous system is hypertrophy of lymphoid tissue in tonsils, alimentary tract, and in the draining lymph nodes; virus has occasionally been recovered from all these sites. The brain shows inflammation with neuronal destruction of the motor cranial nerve nuclei, the reticular formation, the cerebellar roof nuclei, the hypothalamus, the thalamus, and the prefrontal cortex (Bodian, 1959). These situations are affected to some degree even in mild infections; a generalised encephalomyelitis is the rule varied only by the intensity of the destructive process.

Findings in the spinal cord (Fig. 49a, b, c).—Leptomeningitis with abundant lymphocytic infiltration together with a few macrophages and occasional polymorphs is a common finding but is always situated adjacent to regions of myelitis, to which it

Fig. 49

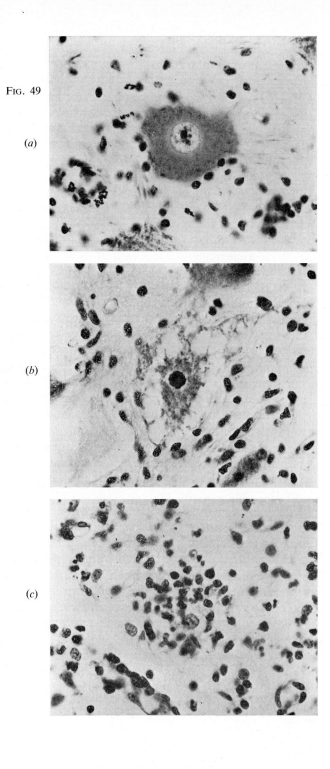

(a)

(b)

(c)

appears to be secondary at the stage of the disease when necropsies are obtained. Baker and Cornwell (1956) found in their series of 50 cases that in 84 per cent of cases the cervical, thoracic and lumbosacral regions were simultaneously affected. The changes affected chiefly the anterior horn but also less often the lateral horn, the base of the posterior horn, and the white matter immediately surrounding the anterior horn. The inflammatory change most constantly seen in the acute stages is a perivascular lymphocytic infiltration which first appears in the anterior horns and in the white matter near the anterior grey commissure, but later spreads to involve the other regions mentioned; when severe the lymphocytic infiltration spreads outside the perivascular space and also may affect the vessel wall with endothelial proliferation causing ischaemia and necrosis. A few polymorphs may be seen in the severe acute cases whose lesions may occasionally be haemorrhagic. Alongside these inflammatory changes are specific alterations in the neurone cell bodies most easily observed in the motoneurones of the anterior horn, and very carefully observed experimentally in monkeys (Bodian, 1959). The first change is a diminution in size of the Nissl bodies and aggregation of the oxychromatin of the nucleus. Chromatolysis then proceeds to a disappearance of the Nissl substance with basophilic cytoplasm, and a shrunken nucleus sometimes with an eosinophilic inclusion body. The neurone dies, the cell body becomes indistinct beneath polymorphs and macrophages, this process being termed neuronophagia. Similar specific changes attributable to virus invasion are seen occasionally in the intermediolateral cells and Clarke's column cells, but can scarcely be recognised in small neurones such as internuncial cells or posterior horn cells. In necropsies on patients dying some time after the acute attack the findings are those of neuronal loss with astrocytic gliosis.

Peripheral nerves and muscles.—The posterior root ganglia may show severe inflammatory changes but the inflammatory changes described in peripheral nerves and muscles are more likely to

FIG. 49 (*see opposite*).—Cellular damage caused by poliomyelitis virus.

(*a*) Infected neurone at the stage of severe diffuse chromatolysis. Note the disappearance of Nissl bodies and the clumping of chromatin in the nucleus.

(*b*) Cytolysis of cell with shrunken nucleus and beaded basophilic border. After complete cytolysis, a punched out, fluid-filled cavity is left which then is reduced by shrinkage and macrophage infiltration.

(*c*) Macrophages and glia cells at site of a completely phagocytosed cell. Gallocyanin stain.

result from the destruction of anterior horn neurones. Thi‹ the conclusion of Bowden (1952), who compared the findin experimental poliomyelitis infections in monkeys with the seq of anterior root section. In acute human cases the muscles degenerating muscle fibres with abnormalities of the teri axons.

In chronic cases, the affected muscle fibres atrophy with spicuous sparing of the muscle spindles. Nerve reinnervation be attempted with branching from intact nerve fibres; this is possible in partially affected muscles, otherwise there is con replacement by fat and fibrous tissue.

Herpes Zoster (Ceinturon de Feu, Gürtelrose, Shingles, Zona`

In herpes zoster there is an inflammation of one or more pos root (or cranial nerve) ganglia with an associated skin eru in the appropriate dermatome. The lesion in the ganglion first described by Felix von Bärensprung (1861–63) and an exc early account is that of Head and Campbell (1900). The : subsequent observations are reviewed by Döring (1955) v detailed account is recommended.

Etiological agent.—Herpes zoster is caused by a virus 210–250 nm by electron microscopy (Rake *et al.*, 1948)) ide or very similar to that causing varicella and apparently inf‹ only for man. The lack of an experimental animal has ham study though human tissue cultures can be inoculated. It is th‹ that the posterior root ganglion is affected by the blood-¶ virus which, travelling neurotropically, then causes the eruption; a minority view is that the pathway is the revers‹ skin being first infected.

Findings in the posterior root ganglion.—The upper cervica the thoracic ganglia are most frequently affected, those c limbs being strangely spared. In my experience one gangl‹ predominantly affected but adjacent ganglia on the same show lesser changes.

Spinal ganglienapoplexie accurately describes the appearai the acute infection; externally there is swelling and congesti the ganglion whilst on cut section a frankly haemorrhagic st seen.

The microscopical appearance is that of haemorrhagic infai sometimes with thrombus in small arterial branches. The : has a central acellular area of complete necrosis surrounded zone of less completely damaged cells mixed with blood and an inflammatory infiltrate mainly of lymphocytes but with some plasma cells and polymorphs. The ganglion cell bodies when not completely necrosed show shrinkage with disappearance of Nissl substance, vacuolation and neuronophagia. Minor inflammatory changes with fibre and myelin loss are seen in the central part of the posterior root and less commonly in the anterior root.

Herpes Zoster Myelitis

The inflammatory lesion seen in the posterior root ganglion may extend into the spinal cord causing a localised area of myelitis with a variable amount of central nervous damage. Clinical cases of spinal cord involvement are relatively common; an early case being that of Broadbent in 1866 (quoted by Wilson, 1954); whilst reporting two cases, Taterka and O'Sullivan (1943) found 42 cases in the literature, and Kendall (1957) was able to record eight personally studied cases in which the spinal cord was involved. The usual finding is a lower motor neurone paralysis affecting muscle groups near the skin eruption. Recovery is slow but usually proceeds to complete functional restoration, consequently necropsy reports are relatively few, but good accounts are those of Lhermitte and Nicolas (1924) and Denny-Brown et al. (1944). In my own experience some perivascular lymphocytic infiltration is always demonstrable in the cord segment related to the affected ganglion; this is usually in relation to the posterior horn but when excessive may spread to involve the anterior horn. Rarer are the cases with long-tract involvement, and three of Kendall's cases were in this category. Wilson (1954) described a case of Brown-Séquard syndrome; a syringomyelia picture was reported by Bruce (1907), whilst a transverse myelitis was present in the case of Gordon and Tucker (1945). All these cases are of a genuine herpes zoster myelitis and are to be distinguished from the categories about to be described.

Infarction in Herpes Zoster (Fig. 50a, b)

There is in herpes zoster a tendency to arterial and venous thrombosis throughout the cardiovascular system (Spillane and White, 1939). Infarction is common in the viscera and in the brain, and it will be recalled that infarction with arterial thrombosis is seen in the actual ganglion lesion. The blood supply of the

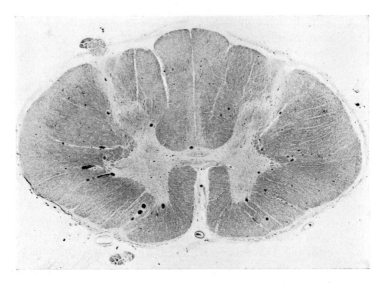

FIG. 50a.—Spinal-cord infarction due to herpes zoster. The picture is of a transverse section at T1 and shows the many dilated and congested vessels. Haematoxylin and eosin ×9.

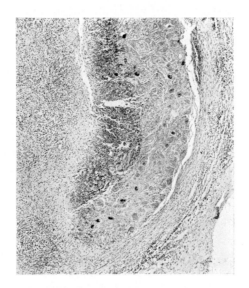

FIG. 50b.—Posterior root ganglion in herpes zoster. The lesion is an acute infarct with haemorrhagic necrosis of the ganglion. Haematoxylin and eosin ×47.

spinal cord is from multiple sources (see Chapter IV), one consequence being a relative immunity to the common causes of vascular occlusion. But when herpes zoster attacks a ganglion whose nerve root is accompanied by a large radicular tributary to the spinal arteries, extensive spinal cord infarction may occur as in the following case:

> An 81-year-old housewife having typical herpes zoster of the right shoulder developed a quadriparesis, trunk paresis and a profound sensory loss below the upper cervical dermatomes. She died four days later after some neurological improvement but marked general deterioration. At necropsy myocardial infarction was present with mural thrombi and pulmonary emboli. The brain showed a recent infarct due to thrombosis of the right anterior cerebral artery. The spinal cord showed early infarction of C2-T1 spinal segments due to vascular occlusion of a radicular tributary accompanying a left cervical root ganglion.

This case report exemplifies the thrombotic tendency in herpes zoster for the heart, brain and spinal cord all showed infarction. The cause of the thrombosis in herpes zoster remains a mystery; possibly there is a direct attack on vascular endothelium.

Secondary or Symptomatic Herpes Zoster

Herpes zoster can secondarily affect sensory ganglia which are directly or indirectly involved by some other disease process. The clinical evidence often suggests the sequence of events, for there are manifestations of the primary disease before the complication of the herpes zoster infection which may localise to the same region of neurological disturbance. The primary disease may be in the spinal cord (syringomyelia, motor neurone disease, tumour, abscess, tabes dorsalis), in the nerve roots and ganglia (trauma, tumours, tuberculous caries, subarachnoid haemorrhage, intrathecal injections) or in the peripheral nerves (alcoholic, arsenical, diabetic or uraemic neuritis, leprosy). Many other diseases have been reported to "attract" a herpes zoster infection and for a full review see Döring (1955). It must be emphasised that in all these cases the herpes zoster infection is quite typical and there is no etiological connection with any of the reported coincidental disease processes. These act, it is thought, merely by damaging the posterior root neurones, either the cell bodies in the ganglion or their axons elsewhere; the result being vulnerability to attack by the zoster virus.

Herpes-B-virus Encephalomyelitis (Herpes Virus Simiae Ence
myelitis)

This interesting endemic disease of monkeys has been occ&
ally reported as a human infection, but always in work&
contact with monkeys. The infection may be the sequel of a m&
bite as in the first reported case of Sabin and Wright (1934), C
of Hummeler *et al.* (1959), and the case of Thomas and Her
(1960), but it may also occur merely from handling the anim
in the case of Sabin (1949), Nagler and Klotz (1958), and I
et al. (1958), or even contact with live extracts of monkey ti
as in Case 2 of Hummeler *et al.* (1959).

Etiological agent and general features.—According to Scott (
the size of the virus particle is approximately 125 nm an&
incubation period 10–20 days. The pathological findings
case are related to the site of inoculation. There may be cel&
around a bite wound with hyperaemia and haemorrhages i
draining lymph nodes, and histological evidence of inflamm&
in lymph nodes and spleen. The central nervous system is aff&
in an ascending sequence with death from involvement o
medulla.

Findings in the spinal cord.—The spinal nerve roots and the
and white matter show a radiculitis and ascending myelitis
inflammatory reaction of lymphocytes and plasma cells is pr
in the spinal nerve roots and perivascularly in the grey and
matter. The white matter has many small foci of necrosis ar
small blood vessels, often amounting to a status spongiosus
grey matter is also profoundly affected with numerous intranu&
inclusion bodies in the neurones. Similar bodies are present i
nuclei of oligodendroglia and of connective tissue cells.

Slow Virus Diseases

The concept of virus diseases with a protracted clinical c&
began with the study in Iceland by Sigurdson (Sigurdson,
and others, of certain neurological diseases of sheep, named
the principal clinical symptom. Thus we have "rida" (tremb
and "visna" (wasting). "Scrapie" (rubbing) is a name by wh
disease of sheep in Europe was well known and this disease is
the subject of intensive investigation.

The interest in these fascinating sheep diseases has
enhanced by comparison with two somewhat similar h&

neurological diseases called kuru and Creutzfeldt-Jakob disease (Lampert *et al.*, 1972). Both of these human diseases have now been transmitted to primates. As with scrapie the transmissible agent has some unusual characteristics but must be classified as a virus.

Kuru

This progressive degenerative disease of the central nervous system has only been recognised in a remote area south of Mount Michael in the Eastern Highlands of New Guinea. The name derives from the prominent symptom of tremor. Kuru means trembling in the language of the Fore tribe who, with a few close neighbours, are the only people known to be affected with the disease. The first full clinical accounts of the condition were those of Zigas and Gajdusek (1957), and Gajdusek and Zigas (1957).

Clinical features.—Kuru affected mainly adult females but also children of both sexes. In the whole susceptible population the incidence was about 1 per cent but in some areas this rose to 10 per cent. These figures appear in the papers quoted above. The incidence of kuru has been declining since the early 1960s and is now less than a third of the figures mentioned. What is very striking is that, for reasons we shall give below, kuru does not now occur in children and the age of the youngest patients seen is gradually increasing.

The clinical course is that of progressive ataxia accompanied by tremor and involuntary movement. The patient becomes bedridden with dysarthria, dysphagia and incontinence of urine and faeces. There is initially a spastic weakness with increased tone and hyperreflexia. Later a flaccid quadriparesis supervenes. The total course to death may be only 3–6 months and rarely exceeds one year; with doubtful exceptions recovery has never been observed.

Pathological findings.—No significant changes have been reported during life in the blood or CSF. At necropsy, specific abnormalities are confined to the central nervous system. The following accounts of the neuropathology have been published: Klatzo *et al.* (1959), Fowler and Robertson (1959), Neumann *et al.* (1964), Kakulas *et al.* (1967).

The brain macroscopically either appears normal or slight atrophy of the frontal lobes and/or the cerebellum may be seen. Microscopically there are widespread neuronal changes with an intense astrocytic gliosis sometimes associated with vacuolation.

These changes are seen throughout the grey matter and are most evident in the pontine nuclei, thalamus, cerebellum and basal ganglia. Extensive secondary degeneration of various tracts leads to a conspicuous loss of the white matter but there is no true demyelination. The white matter degeneration leads to an abundance of microglia but lymphocytic infiltration is uncommon. One prominent feature is the presence of "stellate plaques" containing amyloid-like material and made up, as seen with the electron microscope, of closely packed fibrils. Ultramicroscopic structures within the "stellate plaques" are similar to those found in Pick's disease and in Alzheimer's disease.

When the spinal cord has been examined, striking changes have been seen. The grey matter is affected by a similar neuronal degeneration to that seen in the brain. This appears in the anterior horns as an intense astrocytic gliosis sometimes with vacuolar degeneration. More striking is the white matter loss seen as a severe degeneration of the corticospinal and spinocerebellar tracts. These white matter changes are probably secondary to the neuronal degeneration.

Etiology of kuru.—Kuru can be transmitted to chimpanzees and also to spider, capuchin, squirrel and rhesus monkeys by the inoculation of human brain material from cases of kuru. The experimental disease, which develops after an interval of from 18 months to 3 years, can then be passaged, when the incubation period is reduced to about one year. The pathology of the experimental disease is similar to that of the natural disease except that status spongiosis is common and that the "stellate plaques" are not found. The affected neurones are sometimes swollen with argentophilic intracytoplasmic spheroids. Experimentally, the disease is transmitted by subcutaneous inoculation. In view of the presumed transmission of the natural disease it is interesting that the experimental disease cannot be produced by giving infective brain material by mouth.

The natural disease is thought to affect the Fore tribe because of their strange custom of cannibalism of their dead relatives. This type of cannibalism has now ceased and the incidence of kuru has declined and now only affects adults who were probably infected some years before. It is not clear if the natural disease is acquired by self-inoculation through cuts or abrasions or through the nasal mucosa or conjunctiva. The former selective incidence in women and children can be explained by the custom of these groups preferentially consuming the offal including the brain of the dead person.

Creutzfeldt-Jakob disease

The literature of this interesting but rare sub-acute neurological disease begins with the clinicopathological report of Creutzfeldt (1920). This described a progressive illness in a 22-year-old girl which began with ataxia, progressed to myoclonic movements, spastic paresis and mental disturbance and ended in paralysis, dementia and coma. The pathological changes were those of a widespread neuronal degeneration with neuronophagia and proliferation of astrocytes and gitter cells.

The following year, Jakob (1921) described four cases with a similar course and pathology. Kirschbaum (1968) in an important monograph has gathered the clinical and pathological details of 150 cases. The neuropathological picture and in particular the frequent presence of status spongiosis is very similar to kuru.

It is interesting to read Kirschbaum's concluding speculations about the etiology of this disease for in the same year the first successful transmission experiment (Gibbs et al., 1968) of the disease to a chimpanzee was reported. At least 14 successful experimental transmissions of the human disease have now been reported with an incubation period of 11 to 14 months and a clinical illness in the animal of 1 to $2\frac{1}{2}$ months. Secondary passage to further chimpanzees and transmission to other primates has been achieved (Lampert et al., 1972). These is no doubt that Creutzfeldt-Jakob disease is caused by a virus.

The spinal cord is probably involved in all cases of Creutzfeldt-Jakob disease. The extensive neuronal degeneration of the cerebral cortex results in secondary degeneration of the corticospinal tracts. Spinocerebellar tract degeneration has also been observed (Teichmann, 1935; Jansen and Monrad-Krohn, 1938).

There is also a primary neuronal degeneration which probably affects all the neurone cell groups of the spinal cord although the motor neurones of the anterior horns have been most often mentioned. Neuronophagia occurs and the typical spongiform degeneration may be present but sometimes is not seen.

REFERENCES

BACTERIAL INFECTIONS

ASZKANAZY, C. L. (1952). Sarcoidosis of the central nervous system. *J. Neuropath. exp. Neurol.*, **11**, 392–400.

AYLIFFE, G. A. J., LOWBURY, E. J. L., HAMILTON, J. G. *et al.* (1965). Hospital infection with *Pseudomonas aeruginosa* in neurosurgery. *Lancet*, **2**, 365–369.

BANERJEE, T. and HUNT, W. E. (1972). Spinal cord sarcoidosis. *J. Neurosurg.*, **36**, 490–493.

BEATTIE, F. C. (1970). Disk space abscess simulating disk herniation: report of a case. *Ohio St. med. J.*, **66**, 381–384.

BETTY, M. and LORBER, J. (1963). Intramedullary abscess of the spinal cord. *J. Neurol. Neurosurg. Psychiat.*, **26**, 236–240.

CAMP, W. A. and FRIERSON, J. G. (1962). Sarcoidosis of the central nervous system. A case with postmortem studies. *Arch. Neurol. (Chic.)*, **7**, 432–441.

CHARCOT, J. M. and JOFFROY, A. (1869). Deux cas d'atrophie musculaire progressive. *Arch. Physiol.*, **2**, 354–367, 629–649, 744–760.

CHIARI, H. (1900). Ueber Myelitis suppurativa bei Bronchiektasie. *Z. Heilk.*, **1**, 351–372.

CORBETT, J. J. and ROSENSTERN, B. J. (1971). Pseudomonas meningitis related to spinal anesthesia. *Neurology*, **21**, 946–950.

DAVID, J. P. (1779). Cited in *Medical Classics* (1936), **1**, 278.

ELSBERG, C. A. (1941). *Surgical Diseases of the Spinal Cord, Membranes, and Nerve Roots: symptoms, diagnosis, and treatment*, p. 185. New York: Hoeber.

ERB, W. H. (1892). Ueber syphilitische spinal paralyse. *Neurol. Zbl.*, **11**, 161–168.

FLECHSIG, P. (1876). *Die Leitungsbahnen im Gehirn und Rückenmark des Menschen*. Leipzig: Engelmann.

FROIN, M. G. (1903). Inflammations méningées, avec réaction chromatique fibrineuse et cytologique du liquide céphalo-rachidien. *Gaz. Hôp. (Paris)*, **76**, 1005.

GAGEL, O. (1958). Tabes. In *Handbuch der Speziellen Pathologischen Anatomie und Histologie*, Vol. XIII/2A, pp. 995–1039. Ed. by W. Scholz. Berlin-Göttingen-Heidelberg: Springer.

GELLERSTEDT, N. (1956). Erkrankungen der Dura mater (Pachymeningitis haemorrhagica, Pachymeningitis cervicalis hypertrophica). In *Handbuch der Speziellen Pathologischen Anatomie und Histologie*, Vol. XIII/4, pp. 775–825. Ed. by W. Scholz. Berlin-Göttingen-Heidelberg: Springer.

GINDI, S. EL and FAIRBURN, B. (1969). Intramedullary spinal abscess as a complication of a congenital dermal sinus: case report. *J. Neurosurg.*, **30**, 494–497.

GREENFIELD, J. G. (1963). In *Greenfield's Neuropathology*, 2nd edit., pp. 169 and 172. Ed. by W. Blackwood, W. H. McMenemy, A. Meyer, R. M. Norman and D. S. Russell. London: Edward Arnold.

GRIFFITHS, D. LL., SEDDON, H. J. and ROAF, R. (1956). *Pott's Paraplegia*. London: Oxford University Press.

GUIDETTI, B. and LA TORRE, E. (1967). Hypertrophic spinal pachymeningitis. *J. Neurosurg.*, **26**, 496–503.

HECHST, B. (1931). Beiträge zur Histopathologie der Tabes dorsalis. *Arch. Psychiat. Nervenkr.*, **95**, 207–263.

HEUBNER, O. J. L. (1874). *Die luetische Erkrankung der Hirnarterien nebst allgemeninen Erörterungen zur normalen und pathologischen. Histologie der Arterien*. Leipzig: Vogel.

HOLZMAN, R. S. and BISHKO, F. (1971). Osteomyelitis in heroin addicts. *Ann. intern. Med.*, **75**, 693–696.

KEISER, R. P. and GRIMES, H. A. (1963). Intervertebral disk infections in children. *Clin. Orthop.*, **30**, 163–166.

MCMICHAEL, J. (1945). Spinal tracts subserving micturition in a case of Erb's spinal paralysis. *Brain*, **68**, 162–164.

MANFREDI, M., BOZZAO, L. and FRASCONI, F. (1970). Chronic intramedullary abscess of the spinal cord: case report. *J. Neurosurg.*, **33**, 352–355.

MARTIN, J. P. (1925). Amyotrophic meningo-myelitis. *Brain*, **48**, 153–182.

MONIZ, E. (1925). La pachyméningite spinale hypertrophique et les cavités médullaires. *Rev. Neurol.*, **2**, 433–463.

NAGEOTTE, J. (1903). *Pathogénie du Tabes Dorsal*. Paris: Naud.

NOGUCHI, H. and MOORE, J. W. (1913). A demonstration of *Treponema pallidum* in the brain in cases of general paralysis. *J. exp. Med.*, **17**, 232–238.

PETTE, H. (1924). Weitere klinische und pathologisch-anatomische Beiträge zum Kapitel der Frühlues des Zentralnervensystems. *Z. ges. Neurol. Psychiat.*, **92**, 346–372.

PLUM, F. (1962). Myelitis and myelopathy. In *Clinical Neurology*, Vol. 3, 2nd edit. Ed. by A. B. Baker. New York: Hoeber-Harper.

POTT, P. (1779). *Remarks on Palsy of the Lower Limbs*. London: Johnson.

RICH, A. R. and MCCORDOCK, H. A. (1933). Pathogenesis of tuberculous meningitis. *Bull. Johns Hopk. Hosp.*, **52**, 5–37.

RIFAAT, M., EL-SHAFEI, I., SAMRA, K. and SOROUR, O. (1973). Intramedullary spinal abscess following spinal puncture. *J. Neurosurg.*, **38**, 366–367.

SAHS, A. L. and JOYNT, R. T. (1962). Meningitis. In *Clinical Neurology*, Vol. 2, 2nd edit. Ed. by A. B. Baker. New York: Hoeber-Harper.

SCADDING, J. G. (1967). *Sarcoidosis*. London: Eyre and Spottiswoode.

SCHAUDINN, F. and HOFFMANN, E. (1905). Ueber Spirochaetenbefunde im Lymphdrüsensaft Syphilitischer. *Dtsch. med. Wschr.*, **31**, 711–714.

SCHEIDEGGER, S. (1958). Tuberkulose. In *Handbuch der Speziellen Pathologischen Anatomie und Histologie*, Vol. XIII/2A, pp. 1125–1177. Ed. by W. Scholz. Berlin-Göttingen-Heidelberg: Springer.

SCHLEUSSING, H. (1958). Meningitis ohne die spezifischen Formen. In *Handbuch der Speziellen Pathologischen Anatomie und Histologie*, Vol. XIII/2A, pp. 1–100. Ed. by W. Scholz. Berlin-Göttingen-Heidelberg: Springer.

SEDDON, H. J. (1935). Pott's paraplegia: prognosis and treatment. *Brit. J. Surg.*, **22**, 769–799.

SELBY, R. C. and PILLAY, K. V. (1972). Osteomyelitis and disc infection secondary to *Pseudomonas aeruginosa* in heroin addiction. *J. Neurosurg.*, **37**, 463–466.

SEMINS, H., NUGENT, G. R. and CHOU, S. M. (1972). Intramedullary spinal cord sarcoidosis. *J. Neurosurg.*, **37**, 233–236.

STRÄUSSLER, E. (1958). Die Syphilis des Zentralnervensystem und die progressive Paralyse (quartäre Syphilis). In *Handbuch der Speziellen Pathologischen Anatomie und Histologie*, Vol. XIII/2A, pp. 847–994. Ed. by W. Scholtz. Berlin-Göttingen-Heidelberg: Springer.

WILSON, S. A. K. (1954). *Neurology*, 2nd edit., pp. 510–535. Ed. by A. Ninian Bruce. London: Butterworth.

WIRTH, E. P. and GADO, M. (1973). Incomplete myelographic block with hypertrophic spinal pachymeningitis. *J. Neurosurg.*, **38**, 368–370.

WOLTMAN, H. W. and ADSON, A. W. (1926). Abscess of the spinal cord: report of a case with functional recovery after operation. *Brain*, **49**, 193–206.

WRIGHT, R. L. (1965). Intramedullary spinal cord abscess: report of a case secondary to stab wound with good recovery following operation. *J. Neurosurg.*, **23**, 208–210.

ZEMAN, W. (1958). Morbus Besnier-Boeck-Schaumann. In *Handbuch der Speziellen Pathologischen Anatomie und Histologie*, Vol. XIII/2A, pp. 1100–1112. Ed. by W. Scholz. Berlin-Göttingen-Heidelberg: Springer.

FUNGAL INFECTIONS

ALAJOUANINE, T., HOUDART, R. and DROUHET, E. (1953). Les formes chirurgicales spinales de la torulose; torulome de la queue de cheval. *Rev. neurol.*, **88**, 153–163.

BRUSCHI, M. (1961). Coccidioidomycosis: a primer. *Postgrad. Med.*, **30**, 301–310.

BURSTON, J. and BLACKWOOD, W. (1963). A case of *Aspergillus* infection of the brain. *J. Path. Bact.*, **86**, 225–229.

CARTON, C. A. and MOUNT, L. A. (1951). Neurosurgical aspects of cryptococcosis. *J. Neurosurg.*, **8**, 143–156.

CRAIG, W. M., DOCKERTY, M. B. and HARRINGTON, S. W. (1940). Intravertebral and intrathoracic blastomycoma simulating dumbbell tumour. *Sth. Surg.*, **9**, 759–766.

FITCHETT, M. S. and WEIDMAN, F. D. (1934). Generalised torulosis associated with Hodgkin's disease. *Arch. Path.*, **18**, 225–244.

GOODMAN, J. S., KAUFMAN, L. and KOENIG, M. G. (1971). Diagnosis of cryptococcal meningitis. Value of immunological detection of cryptococcal antigen. *New Engl. J. Med.*, **285**, 434–436.

GREENWOOD, R. C. and VORIS, A. C. (1950). Systemic blastomycosis with spinal cord involvement. *J. Neurosurg.*, **7**, 450–454.

HUGHES, W. T. (1966). Generalised aspergillosis: a case involving the central nervous system. *Amer. J. Dis. Child.*, **112**, 262–265.

IYER, S., DODGE, P. R. and ADAMS, R. D. (1952). Two cases of aspergillus infection of the central nervous system. *J. Neurol. Neurosurg. Psychiat.*, **15**, 152–163.

JACKSON, F. E., KENT, D. and CLARE, F. (1964). Quadriplegia caused by involvement of cervical spine with *Coccidioides immitis*. *J. Neurosurg.*, **21**, 512–515.

JACKSON, I. J., EARLE, K. M. and KURI, J. (1955). Solitary aspergillus granuloma of brain; report of 2 cases. *J. Neurosurg.*, **12**, 53–61.

JUBA, A. (1958). Über eine seltene Mykose (durch Histoplasma capsulatum verursachte Meningoencephalitis) des Zentralnervensystems. *Psychiat. et Neurol. (Basel)*, **135**, 260–268.

LEY, A., JACAS, R. and OLIVERAS, C. (1951). Torula granuloma of the cervical spinal cord. *J. Neurosurg.*, **8**, 327–335.

LITTMAN, M. L., HOROWITZ, P. L. and SWADEY, J. G. (1958). Coccidioidomycosis and its treatment with amphotericin B. *Amer. J. Med.*, **24**, 568–592.

LITTMAN, M. L. and ZIMMERMAN, L. E. (1956). *Cryptococcosis*. New York: Grune and Stratton.

MATHEIS, H. (1960). Die Cryptococcose (Torulose) des Nervensystems. *Dtsch. Z. Nervenheilk.*, **180**, 595–639.

MUKOYAMA, M., GIMPLE, K. and POSER, C. M. (1969). Aspergillosis of the central nervous system. *Neurology*, **19**, 967–974.

NELSON, J. D., BATES, R. and PITCHFORD, A. (1961). Histoplasma meningitis. *Amer. J. Dis. Child.*, **102**, 218–223.

OSMOND, J. D., SCHWEITZER, G., DUNBAR, J. M. and VILLET, W. (1971). Blastomycosis of the spine with paraplegia. *S. African med. J.*, **45**, 431–434.

RAMAMURTHI, B. and ANGULI, V. C. (1954). Intramedullary cryptococcic granuloma of the spinal cord. *J. Neurosurg.*, **11**, 622–624.

RAND, C. W. (1930). Coccidioidal granuloma: report of two cases simulating tumour of spinal cord. *Arch. Neurol. Psychiat. (Chic.)*, **23**, 502–511.

REEVES, D. L., BUTT, E. M. and HAMMACK, R. W. (1941). Torula infection of the lungs and central nervous system. *Arch. intern. Med.*, **68**, 57–79.

SCHULZ, D. M. (1953). Histoplasmosis of the central nervous system. *J. Amer. med. Ass.*, **151**, 549–551.

SCHWARZ, J. and BAUM, G. L. (1951). Blastomycosis. *Amer. J. clin. Path.*, **21**, 999–1029.

SCHWARZ, J. and BAUM, G. L. (1963). Histoplasmosis, 1962. *Arch. intern. Med.*, **111**, 710–718.

SERES, J. L., ONO, H. and BENNER, E. J. (1972). Aspergillosis presenting as spinal cord compression. *J. Neurosurg.*, **36**, 221–224.

SHAPIRO, J. L., LUX, J. J. and SPROFKIN, B. E. (1955). Histoplasmosis of the central nervous system. *Amer. J. Path.*, **31**, 319–335.

SKULTETY, F. M. (1961). Cryptococcic granuloma of the dorsal spinal cord. *Neurology (Minneap.)*, **2**, 1066–1070.

SMITH, F. B. and CRAWFORD, J. S. (1930). Fatal granulomatosis of the central nervous system due to a yeast (torula). *J. Path. Bact.*, **33**, 291–296.

SOLWAY, L. J., KOHAN, M. and PRITZKER, H. G. (1939). A case of disseminated blastomycosis. *Canad. med. Ass. J.*, **41**, 331–336.

WERNER, S. B., PAPPAGIANIS, D., HEINDL, I. and MICKEL, A. (1972). An epidemic of coccidioidomycosis among archaeology students in Northern California. *New Engl. J. Med.*, **286**, 507–512.

WOLSTENHOLME, G. E. W. and PORTER, R. (1968). *Systemic Mycoses.* Ciba Foundation Symposium held in Ibadan, 1967. London: Churchill.

PARASITIC INFESTATIONS

BATSON, O. V. (1940). Function of vertebral veins and their role in spread of metastases. *Ann. Surg.*, **112**, 138–149.

BIRD, A. V. (1964). Acute spinal schistosomiasis. *Neurology (Minneap.)*, **14**, 647–656.

BOGAERT, L. VAN (1958). La trypanosomiase africaine. In *Handbuch der Speziellen Pathologischen Anatomie und Histologie*, Vol. XIII/2A, pp. 1086–1099. Ed. W. Scholz. Berlin-Göttingen-Heidelberg: Springer.

BRÜTT, H. (1931). Über einen erfolgreich operierten Fall von Rückenmarksechinokokkus. *Zbl. Chir.*, **58**, 2066–2070.

BUDZILOVICH, G. N., MOST, H. and FEIGIN, I. (1964). Pathogenesis and latency of spinal cord schistosomiasis. *Arch. Path.*, **77**, 383–388.

BUNNAG, T., COMER, D. S. and PUNYAGUPTA, S. (1970). Eosinophilic myeloencephalitis caused by *Gnathostoma spinigerum*. Neuropathology of nine cases. *J. Neurol. Sci.*, **10**, 419–434.

COSACESCO, A. and VEREANO, D. (1946). Le kyste hydatique épidural primitif. *Presse méd.*, **54**, 871–872.

DAY, H. B. and KENAWY, M. R. (1936). Case of bilharzial myelitis. *Trans. roy. Soc. trop. Med. Hyg.*, **30**, 223–224.

DAZZI, A. and VERGA, P. (1926). Di un raro caso di cisticerco racemoso a localizzazione spinale. *Policlinico (Sez. med.)*, **33**, 65–109.

ESCOBAR, A. and NIETO, D. (1972). Parasitic diseases. In *Pathology of the Nervous System*, Vol. 3, Chap. 180. Ed. by J. Minckler. New York: McGraw-Hill.

FAUST, E. C. (1948). An inquiry into the ectopic lesions in schistosomiasis. *Amer. J. trop. Med.*, **28**, 175–199.

FAUST, E. C. and RUSSEL, P. F. (1957). *Clinical Parasitology*. 6th edit. Philadelphia: Lea and Febiger.

FISCHER, W. (1955). Die parasitären Erkrankungen des Zentralnervensystems und seiner Hüllen. In *Handbuch der Speziellen Pathologischen Anatomie und Histologie*, Vol. XIII/3, pp. 372–412. Ed. by W. Scholz. Berlin-Göttingen-Heidelberg: Springer.

FRENKEL, J. K. (1972). Toxoplasmosis. In *Pathology of the Nervous System*, Vol. 3, Chap. 181. Ed. by J. Minckler. New York: McGraw-Hill.

GAMA, R. A. C. and MARQUES DE SA, J. (1945). Esquistossomose medular; granulomas produzidos por ovas de *Schistosoma mansoni* comprimindo a medula, epicone, cone e cauda equina. *Arch. Neuro-psiquiat. (S. Paulo)*, **3**, 337–346.

HERSKOWITZ, A. (1972). Spinal cord involvement with *Schistosoma mansoni*. *J. Neurosurg.*, **36**, 494–498.

HESKETH, K. T. (1965). Cysticercosis of the dorsal cord. *J. Neurol. Neurosurg. Psychiat.*, **28**, 445–448.

HOFF, H. and SHABY, J. A. (1939). Nervous and mental manifestations of bilharziasis and their treatment. *Trans. roy. Soc. trop. Med. Hyg.*, **33**, 107–111.

HUTTON, P. W. and HOLLAND, J. T. (1960). Schistosomiasis of the spinal cord; report of a case. *Brit. med. J.*, **2**, 1931–1933.

KAHN, P. (1972). Cysticercosis of the central nervous system with amyotrophic lateral sclerosis: case report and review of the literature. *J. Neurol. Neurosurg. Psychiat.*, **35**, 81–87.

KORBSCH, H. (1932). Über Ruckenmarkscysticerkose. *Dtsch. Z. Chir.*, **237**, 779–784.

MACIEL, Z., COELHO, B. and ABATH, G. (1954). Myélite schistosomique due au *S. mansoni*; étude anatomo-clinique. *Rev. neurol.*, **91**, 241–259.

MANUELIDIS, E. E. (1972). Trypanosomal encephalitides. In *Pathology of the Nervous System*, Vol. 3, Chap. 183. Ed. by J. Minckler. New York: McGraw-Hill.

MÜLLER, H. R. and STENDER, A. (1930). Bilharziose des Rückenmarkes unter dem Bilde einer Myelitis dorsolumbalis transversa completa. *Arch. Schiffs.-u. Tropenhyg.*, **34**, 527–538.

ODEKU, E. L., LUCAS, A. O. and RICHARD, D. R. (1968). Intramedullary spinal cord schistosomiasis. *J. Neurosurg.*, **29**, 417–423.

OH, S. J. (1968). Spinal paragonimiasis. *J. Neurol. Sci.*, **6**, 125–140.

OH, S. J. (1969). Cerebral and spinal paragonimiasis. A histopathological study. *J. Neurol. Sci.*, **9**, 205–236.

PEPLER, W. J. and LOMBAARD, C. M. (1958). Spinal cord granuloma due to *Schistosoma haematobium*: report of one case. *J. Neuropath. exp. Neurol.*, **17**, 656–659.

POPOV, N. A. and UMEROW, B. T. (1935). Echinococcus der Wirbelsäule und des Rückenmarks. *Dtsch. Z. Nervenheilk.*, **137**, 187–196.

ROSENBLATH. (1913). Ein Fall von Cysticerkenmeningitis mit vorwiegender Beteiligung des Rückenmarks. *Dtsch. Z. Nenrveheilk.*, **46**, 113–126.

ROSS, G. L., NORCROSS, J. W. and HORRAX, G. (1952). Spinal cord involvement by *Schistosoma mansoni*. *New Engl. J. Med.*, **246**, 823–826.

SAWITZ, W. G. (1956). *Medical Parasitology*. New York: McGraw-Hill.

SCHEIDEGGER, S. (1958a). Malaria. In *Handbuch der Speziellen Pathologischen Anatomie und Histologie*, Vol. XIII/2A, pp. 1113–1124. Ed. by W. Scholz. Berlin-Göttingen-Heidelberg: Springer.

SCHEIDEGGER, S. (1958b). Pilzerkrankungen. In *Handbuch der Speziellen Pathologischen Anatomie und Histologie*, Vol. XIII/2A, pp. 1178–1221. Ed. by W. Scholz. Berlin-Göttingen-Heidelberg: Springer.

SENNARA, H. (1969), Bilharzial paraplegia: report of a case. *J. Bone Jt Surg.*, **51B**, 132–134.

WAKEFIELD, G. S., CARROLL, J. D. and SPEED, D. E. (1962). Schistosomiasis of the spinal cord. *Brain*, **85**, 535–552.

VIRUS DISEASES

BADHAM, J. (1834). Paralysis in childhood; four remarkable cases of suddenly induced paralysis in the extremities, occurring in children, without any apparent cerebral or cerebro-spinal lesion. *Lond. med. Gaz.*, **17**, 215–218.

BAKER, A. B. and CORNWELL, S. (1956). Poliomyelitis. XV. The spinal cord. *Arch. Neurol. Psychiat. (Chic.)*, **61**, 185–206.

BÄRENSPRUNG, F. W. F. VON (1861–63). Die Gürtelkrankheit. *Ann. Charite-Krankenh. zu Berlin*, **9**, (2) 40–128, **10**, (1) 37–53, **11** (2) 96–116.

BERNTSEN, C. A. and STEVENSON, L. D. (1953). Human rabies. *J. Neuropath. exp. Neurol.*, **12**, 169–185.

BIELING, R. and POETSCHKE, G. (1958). Allgemeine Pathogenese der

Viruskrankheiten des Zentralnervensystems. In *Handbuch der Speziellen Pathologischen Anatomie und Histologie*, Vol. XIII/2A, pp. 101–161. Ed. by W. Scholz. Berlin-Göttingen-Heidelberg: Springer.

BISSERU, B. (1972). *Rabies*. London: Heinemann.

BODIAN, D. (1959). In *Viral and Rickettsial Infections of Man*, 3rd edit., pp. 479–498. Ed. by T. M. Rivers and F. L. Horsfall. Philadelphia: Lippincott.

BODIAN, D., MORGAN, I. M. and HOWE, H. A. (1949). Differentiation of types of poliomyelitis viruses. III. The grouping of fourteen strains into three basic immunological types. *Amer. J. Hyg.*, **49**, 234–245.

BOGAERT, L. VAN (1958). Poliomyélite antérieure aigue (Maladie de Heine-Medin). In *Handbuch der Speziellen Pathologischen Anatomie und Histologie*, Vol. XIII/2A, pp. 244–297. Ed. by W. Scholz. Berlin-Göttingen-Heidelberg: Springer.

BOWDEN, R. E. M. (1952). Some recent studies of skeletal muscle in anterior poliomyelitis and other neuromuscular disorders in man and the experimental animal. *Poliomyelitis: papers and discussion presented at the 2nd Internat. Conf.*, pp. 95–99. Philadelphia: Lippincott.

BRUCE, A. (1907). Unusual sequela of herpes zoster (? posterior poliomyelitis). *Rev. Neurol. Psychiat.*, **5**, 885–896.

CHARCOT, J. M. and JOFFROY, A. (1870). Cas de paralysie infantile spinale avec lésions des cornes antérieures de la substance grise de la moelle épinière. *Arch. physiol. norm. et path.*, **3**, 134–152.

CREUTZFELDT, H. G. (1920). Über eine eigenartige herdformige Erkrankung des Zentralnervensystems. *Z. ges. Neurol. Psychiat.*, **57**, 1–18.

DENNY-BROWN, D., ADAMS, R. D. and FITZGERALD, P. J. (1944). Pathologic features of herpes zoster. *Arch. Neurol. Psychiat. (Chic.)*, **51**, 216–231.

DÖRING, G. (1955). Zoster. In *Handbuch der Speziellen Pathologischen Anatomie und Histologie*, Vol. XIII/5, pp. 291–312. Ed. by W. Scholz. Berlin-Göttingen-Heidelberg: Springer.

ELFORD, W. J., GALLOWAY, I. A. and PERDRAU, J. R. (1935). The size of the virus of poliomyelitis as determined by ultrafiltration analysis. *J. Path. Bact.*, **40**, 135–140.

FOWLER, M. and ROBERTSON, E. G. (1959). Observations on kuru. III. Pathological features in five cases. *Aust. Ann. Med.*, **8**, 16–26.

GAJDUSEK, D. C. and ZIGAS, V. (1957). Degenerative disease of the central nervous system in New Guinea. The endemic occurrence of "Kuru" in the native population. *New Engl. J. Med.*, **257**, 974–978.

GALLOWAY, I. A. and ELFORD, W. J. (1936). Size of virus of rabies ("fixed" strain) by ultrafiltration analysis. *J. Hyg. (Lond.)*, **36**, 532–535.

GIBBS, C. J., JR, GAJDUSEK, D. C., ASHER, D. M. *et al.* (1968). Creutzfeldt-Jakob disease (spongiform encephalopathy): transmission to the chimpanzee. *Science*, **161**, 388–389.

GOLDWASSER, R. A. and KISSLING, R. E. (1958). Fluorescent antibody staining of street and fixed virus antigens. *Proc. Soc. exp. Biol. (N.Y.)*, **98**, 219–223.

GORDON, I. R. S. and TUCKER, JOYCE F. (1945). Lesions of the central nervous system in herpes zoster. *J. Neurol. Neurosurg. Psychiat.*, **8**, 40–46.

HEAD, H. and CAMPBELL, A. W. (1900). The pathology of herpes zoster and its bearing on sensory localisation. *Brain*, **23**, 353–523.

HEINE, J. (1840). *Beobachtungen über Lähmungszustände der unteren Extremitäten und deren Behandlung.* Stuttgart: Köhler.

HORÁNYI-HECHST, B. (1935). Zur Histopathologie der menschlichen Poliomyelitis acuta anterior. *Dtsch. Z. Nervenheilk.*, **137**, 1–54.

HUMMELER, K., DAVIDSON, W. L., HENLE, W., LA BOCCETTA, A. C. and RUSH, H. G. (1959). Encephalomylitis due to infection with herpes virus simiae (Herpes B virus). A report of two fatal laboratory-acquired cases. *New Engl. J. Med.*, **261**, 64–68.

HURST, E. W. and PAWAN, J. L. (1931). An outbreak of rabies in Trinidad. *Lancet*, **2**, 622–628.

HURST, E. W. and PAWAN, J. L. (1932). A further account of the Trinidad outbreak of acute rabic myelites. *J. Path. Bact.*, **35**, 301–321.

JAKOB, A. (1921). Über eigenartige Erkrankungen des Zentralnervensystems mit bemerkenswertem anatomischen Befunde (spastische Pseudosklerose-Encephalomyelopathie) mit disseminierten Degenerationsherden. *Dtsch. Z. Nervenheilk.*, **70**, 132–146.

JANSEN J., and MONRAD-KROHN, G. H. (1938). Über die Creutzfeldt-Jakobsche Krankheit. *Z. ges. Neurol. Psychiat.*, **163**, 670–704.

KAKULAS, B. A., LECOURS, A. R. and GAJDUSEK, D. C. (1967). Further observations on the pathology of kuru. *J. Neuropath. exp. Neurol.*, **26**, 85–97.

KENDALL, D. (1957). Motor complications of Herpes Zoster. *Brit. med. J.*, **2**, 616–618.

KIRSCHBAUM, W. R. (1968). *Jakob-Creutzfeldt Disease.* New York: American Elsevier.

KLATZO, I., GAJDUSEK, D. C. and ZIGAS, V. (1959). Pathology of kuru disease. *J. Neuropath. exp. Neurol.*, **18**, 335–336.

LAMPERT, P. W., GAJDUSEK, D. C. and GIBBS, C. J. (1972). Subacute spongiform virus encephalopathies. *Amer. J. Path.*, **68**, 625–652.

LANDSTEINER, K. and POPPER, E. (1909). Uebertragung der Poliomyelitis acuta auf Affen. *Z. Immun.-Forsch.*, **2**, 377–390.

LASSEN, H. C. A. (1962). Paralytic human rabies in Greenland. *Lancet*, **1**, 247–249.

LHERMITTE, J. and NICOLAS. (1924). Les lésions spinales du zona: La myélite zostérienne. *Rev. neurol.*, **1**, 361–364.

NAGLER, F. P. and KLOTZ, M. (1958). A fatal B-virus infection in a person subject to recurrent herpes labialis. *Canad. med. Ass. J.*, **79**, 743–745.

NEGRI, A. (1903). Beitrag zum Studium der Aetiologie der Tollwut. *Z. Hyg. Infekt.-Kr.*, **43**, 507–528.

NEUMANN, M. A., GAJDUSEK, D. C. and ZIGAS, V. (1964). Neuropathologic findings in exotic neurologic disorders among natives of the highlands of New Guinea. *J. Neuropath. exp. Neurol.*, **23**, 486–507.

NIEBERG, K. C. and BLUMBERG, J. M. (1972). Viral encephalitides. In *Pathology of the Nervous System*, Vol. 3, Chap. 169. Ed. by J. Minckler. New York: McGraw-Hill.

NOORDAM, A. L. (1963). Rabies in Amsterdam. *Med. Contact (Amst.)*, **18**, 415–418, 438–440, 456–457.

PAUL, J. M. (1829). Case of paralysis occurring in a child, and attended with anomalous symptoms. *N. Amer. med. surg. J.*, **8**, 70.

PIERCE, E. C., PEIRCE, J. D. and HULL, R. N. (1958). B. virus: Its current significance. Description and diagnosis of a fatal human infection. *Amer. J. Hyg.*, **68**, 242–250.

RAKE, G., BLANK, H., CORIELL, L. L., NAGLER, F. P. O. and SCOTT, T. F. M. (1948). The relationship of varicella and herpes zoster: electron microscopy studies. *J. Bact.*, **56**, 293–303.

SABIN, A. B. (1949). Fatal B-virus encephalomyelitis in a physician working with monkeys. *J. clin. Invest.*, **28**, 808.

SABIN, A. B. and WRIGHT, A. M. (1934). Acute ascending myelitis following a monkey bite, with the isolation of a virus capable of reproducing the disease. *J. exp. Med.*, **59**, 115–134.

SCHÜKRI, I. and SPATZ, H. (1925). Ueber die anatomischen veränderungen bei der menschlichen Lyssa und ihre Beziehingen zu denen der Encephalitis epidemica. *Z. ges. Neurol. Psychiat.*, **97**, 627–650.

SCOTT, T. F. M. (1959). In *Viral and Rickettsial Infections of Man*, 3rd edit., pp. 769. Ed. by T. M. Rivers and F. L. Horsfall, Philadelphia: Lippincott.

SELLERS, T. F. (1927). A new method for staining Negri bodies of rabies. *Amer. J. publ. Hlth*, **17**, 1080–1081.

SIGURDSON, V. (1954). Observations on three slow infections of sheep. *Brit. vet. J.*, **110**, 255–270, 307–322, 341–354.

SPILLANE, J. D. and WHITE, P. D. (1939). Herpes zoster and angina pectoris. *Brit. Heart J.*, **1**, 291–302.

SÜKRÜ-AKSEL, I. (1958). Pathologische Anatomie der Lyssa. In *Handbuch der Speziellen Pathologischen Anatomie und Histologie*, Vol.

XIII/2A, pp. 417–435. Ed. by W. Scholz. Berlin-Göttingen-Heidelberg: Springer.

TATERKA, J. H. and O'SULLIVAN, M. E. (1943). Motor complications of herpes zoster. *J. Amer. med. Ass.*, **122**, 737–739.

TEICHMANN, E. (1935). Über einen der amyotrophischen Lateralsclerose nahestehenden Krankheitsprozen mit psychischen Symptomen. *Z. ges. Neurol. Psychiat.*, **154**, 32–44.

THOMAS, E. and HENSCHEL, E. (1960). Über die Herpes-B-virus-Myelitis und Encephalitis beim Menschen. *Dtsch. Z. Nervenheilk.*, **181**, 494–516.

UNDERWOOD, M. (1789). Debility of the Lower extremities. In *A Treatise on the Diseases of Children*, Vol. 2, 2nd edit., pp. 53–57. London: Printed for J. Mathews.

WHITTY, C. W. M., HUGHES, J. T. and MacCALLUM, F. O. (1969). *Virus Diseases and the Nervous System.* Oxford: Blackwell.

WICKMAN, I. (1913). *Acute Poliomyelitis (Heine–Medin Disease);* authorized English translation by Dr. W. J. M. A. Maloney. Monograph Series No. 16, New York: Journal of Nervous and Mental Disorders Publishing Co.

WILSON, S. A. K. (1954). In *Neurology*, 2nd edit., pp. 777–778. Ed. by A. N. Bruce. London: Butterworth.

ZIGAS, V. and GAJDUSEK, D. C. (1957). Kuru: clinical study of a new syndrome resembling paralysis agitans in natives of the Eastern Highlands of Australian New Guinea. *Med. J. Aust.*, **2**, 745–754.

CHAPTER VII

DISORDERS OF THE SPINE

The spinal cord may be involved by various disorders of the spinal column and these form such a heterogeneous collection that it is convenient to consider them together in one chapter. The anatomical features of the spinal column are of considerable importance in the understanding of its disorders, but for details the reader is referred to the larger anatomical treatises. The remarkable feature about the spinal column is the protection it affords to its contents by the bony canal whilst at the same time preserving flexibility by its articulative structure. It is worth emphasising that the cervical and upper thoracic part of the spinal column are more flexible and slighter in construction than the lower thoracic and lumbosacral parts, which become progressively more massive as one proceeds caudally. Although the variety of disorders of the spine is considerable, one common recurrent mechanism of spinal cord damage is that of pressure exerted on the spinal cord, and this factor is so important that it merits special consideration. An account of the experimental work on spinal cord compression and the mechanism of its action in human diseases will be found in Chapter X.

DEVELOPMENTAL ABNORMALITIES OF THE SPINAL CANAL

There are many different types of developmental abnormalities of the spinal canal, which cause or are associated with spinal cord dysfunction, but none are particularly common except *spina bifida*, which is dealt with in Chapter II. A group of inter-related developmental disorders in the region of the foramen magnum are frequently associated with neurological disturbance. They will be described under their descriptive names but it must be borne in mind that they frequently coexist. The best known, although not of common occurrence, is the Klippel–Feil syndrome in which there is a midline cleft of the occipital bone and the cervical vertebral laminae with a varying degree of maldevelopment of the cervical vertebral bodies, some of which may be fused.

The neck is shortened and there may be webbing between the head and shoulders. Associated with these bony abnormalities but not necessarily caused by them are disturbances of power and sensibility in the upper limbs. This condition and the closely related abnormality of iniencephaly are dealt with in Chapter II. Here we shall deal with the various developmental abnormalities found at the upper end of the spine and in that part of the skull which surrounds the foramen magnum. The papers of McRae (1953), Spillane *et al.* (1957), Bharucha and Dastur (1964) and of Dastur *et al.* (1965) give observations based on clinical and radiological examinations on these cases. These developmental abnormalities will be subdivided as follows: atlas fusion, platybasia and basilar invagination, and chronic atlanto-axial dislocation. The condition of achondroplasia will be described separately.

Atlas Fusion

McRae (1953), in describing the radiological features of over 100 cases with bony abnormalities in this region, found atlas fusion in 28. In these cases the atlas was partially or completely united by bone to the ring around the foramen magnum. The narrowing of the spinal cord depended on the position of the odontoid process which varied in its length and angulation. In McRae's cases, neurological signs were always present when the anteroposterior diameter of the canal (behind the odontoid process) was narrowed to 19 mm or less. Atlas fusion is nearly always a developmental defect and it may be associated with fusion of other cervical vertebrae.

Bharucha and Dastur (1964) found occipitalisation of the atlas in 23 out of their 40 cases.

Platybasia and Basilar Invagination

Platybasia means flattening of the base of the skull and the degree of this abnormality is measured radiologically by the angle formed between the anterior cranial fossa and the clivus. Normally the angle is 135° or less and when it greatly exceeds this, platybasia is said to be present. *Basilar invagination* or *basilar impression* means an upward bulging of the margins of the foramen magnum and this may be a congenital developmental abnormality or may be secondary to a softened state of the bone of the posterior cranial fossa. Bharucha and Dastur found in their 40 developmental cases that basilar invagination was present in 6. The commonest cause of the secondary type is Paget's disease but the syndrome has followed rickets, and various osteomalacic states. The congenital type is often seen with a hereditary background (Bull *et al.*, 1955) and, as with all these malformations, allied conditions such as cervical vertebral fusion are frequently present. The serious consequence of basilar invagination is angulation of the spinal canal and again the narrowest part is behind the odontoid process. In a case described by Greenfield the spinal cord was narrowed to a flattened ribbon only 2 mm in its anteroposterior diameter.

Separation of the Odontoid Process

In McRae's cases the odontoid process was separate from the axis in 11 out of 100 instances of his series of developmental disorders. Two of his patients, both children, appeared to have congenital malformations. In the adult cases, it was difficult to ascribe the separation with certainty either to a congenital malformation or to an old non-united fracture of the odontoid process. These cases may show signs of cord compression but this may take years to be fully manifest as in the case of Bachs *et al.* (1955).

Chronic Atlanto-axial Dislocation

McRae found this state in 6 out of 100 of his cases. The atlas vertebra was displaced anteriorly in relation to the axis and there was little movement either between atlas and axis or between atlas and skull. Three of McRae's cases were of congenital origin, having associated defects such as spina bifida and fused cervical vertebrae. There was no association with atlas fusion, platybasia, or basilar invagination. Neurological symptoms and signs were present in three cases but in all six cases the spinal canal was angulated and narrowed in its anteroposterior diameter.

The account of Dastur *et al.* (1965) describes the clinical and necropsy findings in six cases of medullospinal compression caused by atlanto-axial dislocation, two cases having odontoid process separation as described above. One interesting feature of the cases was the sudden development of haematomyelia following an otherwise successful decompressive operation.

Achondroplasia

This is a completely different disorder from those just described. The defect is one of endochondral ossification and results in dwarfism. The neurological disturbances are secondary to spinal deformity and good accounts are to be found in the reports of Freund (1933), Vogl and Osborne (1949), Spillane (1952), Epstein and Malis (1955), and Duvoisin and Yahr (1962). The structural changes in the spine were described by Donath and Vogl (1925). As in the long bones the longitudinal growth of the vertebral bodies, neural arches, spinal laminae and spinal pedicles is retarded but, whilst these structures remain short, they thicken considerably due to increased periosteal bone formation. This bony thickening considerably narrows the spinal canal which may also be angulated by a severe thoracolumbar kyphosis, which is common in achondroplasia. These structural changes lead, in some cases, to a slowly progressive neurological syndrome due to compression of the spinal cord and cauda equina.

TOXIC AND METABOLIC DISORDERS OF THE SPINE

Fluorosis (Chronic Fluorine Intoxication)

This is a condition in which there is accumulation in the body of excessive fluoride ion usually by the ingestion, over a long period of a water supply containing an excessive amount of fluorine. The condition occurs in endemic form in certain areas of the world and has been reported (Singh et al., 1963) from several parts of India, and by other observers from China, Japan, South Africa, North Africa, Argentine, Persian Gulf, Saudi Arabia, United States, Canada and Europe. The effects on the body of excessive fluoride are protean but the effect on the spinal cord and its nerve roots, with which we are concerned here, is secondary to changes in the spine. The effect of excessive fluoride on the skeleton is to cause extensive mineralisation with bony enlargement and irregular bone deposition in soft tissues. The spinal canal is narrowed and there is pressure on the spinal cord or its nerve roots. Neurological complications of fluorosis only occur in the most extreme forms of the intoxication and have only been described in India. The earliest report was that of Shortt et al. (1937) and there have been subsequent accounts by Siddiqui (1955) and Singh et al. (1961, 1963).

Many years (30–40 according to Shortt *et al.*) of ingestion of fluorides were thought necessary before skeletal fluorosis develops. Consequently the disease is only common in the elderly. However Teotia *et al.* (1971) have described the condition, again from India, in children.

Clinical features.—These are of both a radiculopathy and a myelopathy. Dysaesthesiae and pain are experienced in areas corresponding to certain nerve roots and there may be localised weakness and wasting of muscles. The myelopathy causes a progressive paraparesis of spastic type together with sensory loss, often below a distinct sensory level. The cerebrospinal fluid protein has been reported elevated and myelograms may demonstrate a spinal block. X-rays readily establish the diagnosis as the skeletal radiological changes are distinctive and characteristic.

Pathological findings.—At necropsy the bones, including the spine, show osteosclerosis which, in a case with myelopathy is of a gross degree. The spinal canal is severely narrowed in an irregular manner (Singh *et al.*, 1963) with distortion of the lumen into a narrow slit. The intervertebral foramina are narrowed or obliterated. Consequent on these bony changes the spinal cord and its nerve roots are compressed. The whole syndrome has many similarities to that produced by cervical spondylosis, but the progression of myelopathy due to fluorosis is rapid and the final structural deformity is greater in this disease.

Disorders of Bone Metabolism (Fig. 51)

The commonest disorder of bone metabolism is probably Paget's disease (osteitis deformans) which is well known to cause spinal cord compression. There are many reports from which I have selected those of Wyllie (1923), Elkington (1939), Turner (1940), Teng *et al.* (1951), and Brenner (1962). In Paget's disease the affected bones enlarge and in the spine this causes a general reduction of the lumen of the spinal canal. Bony projections from the posterior surfaces of the vertebral bodies may further narrow the spinal canal. The bones in Paget's disease, although enlarged, are softer than normal and severe kyphosis may occur. In hypoparathyroidism and the similar condition pseudohypoparathyroidism abnormal bone formation is an important part of the syndrome and this may cause spinal cord compression as in the case of Cullen and Pearce (1964). Spinal cord compression has also been reported due to bony overgrowth in a case of vitamin

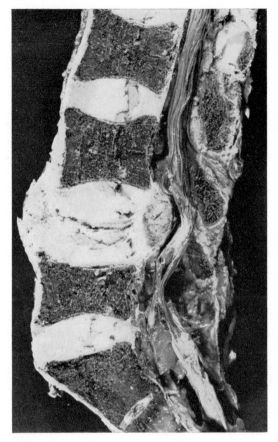

FIG. 51.—Sagittally sawn specimen of the lumbosacral spine from a case of osteo-porosis. Note the collapse of the fourth lumbar vertebra and the pressure on the roots of the cauda equina.

D-resistant rickets (Dugger and Vandiver, 1966). Albright's syn-drome (polyostotic fibrous dysplasia) is a developmental abnor-mality of bone in which multiple tumour-like malformations occur and these, in the case of Teng *et al.* (1951), caused para-plegia.

The inborn errors of lipoid metabolism affect the spinal column by causing its expansion and replacement by abnormal storage material and it is conceivable that, in any of these con-ditions, disturbances of the spinal cord may occur. Raynor (1962) described spinal cord compression in a case of Gaucher's disease which had caused the collapse of vertebral bodies and angulation of the spine. Kennedy *et al.* (1973) described the case of one of two sisters suffering from mucopolysaccharidosis who developed a progressive paraparesis due to compression of the cervical spinal cord. The cause of the compression appeared to be ligamentous thickening together with bony stenosis of the spinal canal. The importance of this neurological complication is that decompressive laminectomy can reverse the paraparesis.

DEGENERATIVE DISEASES OF THE SPINE

A variety of degenerative conditions affect the intervertebral discs, the intervertebral joints, and the vertebrae of the spinal column, but only some of these conditions cause an effect on the spinal cord. First we shall describe the so-called prolapsed intervertebral disc and then the effect of spondylosis (mainly of the cervical region) on the spinal cord. These two conditions are very much more common than cases in which the spinal cord is damaged by joint diseases such as rheumatoid arthritis and ankylosing spondylitis.

PROLAPSED INTERVERTEBRAL DISC

One of the earliest accounts of this condition was that of Luschka (1858) and another important report was that of Kocher (1896). There are many other earlier reports but these are difficult to interpret owing to the confusion between traumatic disc rupture and the degenerative condition of spondylosis. Middleton and Teacher (1911) and Goldthwait (1911) described cases that were clearly those where prolapse of intervertebral disc material occurred after trauma. For a full review of the development of our knowledge of the subject the reader is referred to Mixter (1951).

Clinical history.—Protrusion of the intervertebral disc is a disease of early adult life and in about half the cases there is a definite history of some sort of injury or strain immediately preceding the onset of the symptoms. Although the condition can occur in any part of the spine it commonly involves the lower three lumbar discs and consequently affects the spinal nerve roots more often than the spinal cord itself. The clinical syndromes resulting are too well known for it to be necessary to describe them here.

Pathology of the intervertebral disc.—The basis of the condition is a herniation of the fluid nucleus pulposus through a weakened or torn part of the annulus fibrosus. The annulus fibrosus is thinner in its posterior region and because of this the rupture is usually in a backward direction. The rupture may also occur directly into the bone of the vertebral body causing a lesion called a Schmorl's node. The protruding portion of the nucleus pulposus enters the spinal canal either as a single sessile mass or in several separate portions. Sometimes the outer fibres of the annulus fibrosus do not rupture but bulge into the spinal canal with their contained portions of the nucleus pulposus. The posterior longitudinal ligament also restrains the bulging of this material into the spinal canal and as this ligament is more developed centrally the herniations of material are usually directed laterally on one or both sides.

Findings in the spinal cord.—Involvement of the spinal cord is confined to cervical and thoracic protrusions which are rather rare and cases with necropsy findings are infrequently encountered. My experience is confined to a single case of a thoracic disc protrusion with myelopathy. The meninges were thickened and indented by the disc protrusion The spinal cord was flattened and deformed on its anterior aspect by a pressure cavity 1 cm transversely, 1.7 cm from above down and 0.6 cm deep. This cavity was centred on the tenth thoracic cord segment. The histological sections showed an old gliotic scar situated mainly in the anterior and lateral part of the right lateral white column. The irregular shape and asymmetry of the cord lesion suggested some type of traumatic compression. Despite the extensive cord damage, the nerve fibres of the posterior columns and of both lateral corticospinal tracts were largely intact and appeared to traverse the damaged spinal cord segment.

CERVICAL SPONDYLOSIS

This is a small part of a generalised disease of the spine called *Spinal osteophytosis* or *Spondylosis deformans*. The disease is so common that it must have been observed in the earliest necropsy examinations performed. The many early accounts of the spinal condition are reported under a confusing number of synonyms and reviews of the more important papers of this wealth of literature have been made by Brain *et al.* (1952), Clarke and Robinson (1956) and Sandler (1961). As in many diseases of the spine, we are indebted for a clear account of pathology to Schmorl (Schmorl and Junghans, 1959). Schmorl made a detailed study of diseases of the spine, which was based on the meticulous examination of a consecutive series of autopsies at Dresden. He was particularly interested in diseases of the intervertebral discs and separated for the first time many confused diseases of bone, intervertebral joints, and intervertebral discs. Schmorl proposed the name *Spondylosis deformans* for this condition with which he was familiar. He insisted that the disease was a primary degenerative process and explained in detail how the bony, cartilaginous and fibrous tissue overgrowth takes place.

Structural Changes in Spondylosis (Fig. 52*a*, *b*, *c*)

The anatomical and pathological features of spondylosis are best seen in a sagittal section of the spinal column. The vertebral bodies are normally separated by a certain width of intervertebral disc; the amount varies in different regions of the spine. In spondylosis, the disc space has become narrow and the disc bulges centrifugally in all directions. Above and below the outwardly moved portion of disc are the osteophytes. The osteophyte consists of new bone formation and this structure together with new cartilage and fibrous tissue is all-important in spondylosis. All these tissues make up the bulge which, when directed posteriorly, encroaches on the spinal canal. The effect is far greater than would be produced merely by movement outwards of the intervertebral disc. This osteophyte formation does not occur in disc prolapse, but such misplaced disc material may calcify.

Difference from Prolapsed Intervertebral Disc

The prolapsed intervertebral disc protrusion is a herniation of fluid nucleus pulposus through a breach in the surrounding annulus fibrosus. The protrusion occurs suddenly, often after trauma, and the episode usually occurs in early adult life. The nucleus pulposus herniation may partially return but usually is permanent; then the herniated material becomes lifeless with necrosis and calcification. There is no osteophyte formation and the narrowing of the spinal canal, if any, must be small. Even if the whole of the nucleus pulposus herniated, it has been estimated that only about 0.7 ml of material would be involved. These cases of prolapse of the intervertebral disc have quite different structural changes from those found in spondylosis. In spondylosis there is no herniation of the nucleus pulposus and even the word protrusion is ambiguous since there is no protrusion out

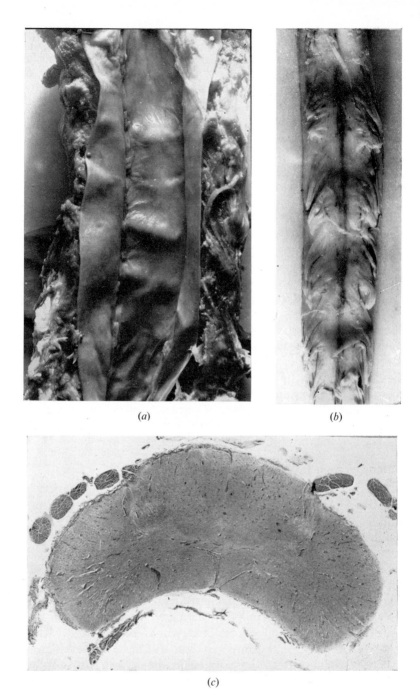

(a)

(b)

(c)

Fig. 52

of the centre of the disc, only a spreading outwards of the whole disc combined with bony, cartilaginous, and fibrous overgrowth.

The Mechanism of the Development of Spondylosis

About one-quarter of the vertebral column in the normal adult is made up of the intervertebral discs and these are subjected to considerable pressure. The pressure within the disc, measured by lumbar discometry (Nachemson and Morris, 1963), is very much raised from the recumbency figures when the individual is standing, and is particularly high when lifting heavy weights. This varying pressure is borne by the discs, whose remarkable feature is elasticity, particularly of the fluid nucleus pulposus. As a senile degenerative change, the disc becomes less fluid and less elastic and the force, exerted between one vertebra and the next, is absorbed by a relatively rigid non-elastic structure. The result is a gradual spreading out of the disc beyond the margins of the vertebral body. As the intervertebral disc spreads outwards, so the periosteum above and below is moved outward. This outwardly moved periosteum causes new bone formation resulting in the osteophyte. A histological section will show the true extent of the osteophytosis, but the spondylotic bulge is further added to by displaced cartilage and often newly formed connective tissue.

Neurological Complications of Spondylosis

Although spondylosis occurs at all levels of the spine, neurological complications are almost entirely due to spondylosis affecting the cervical spine. Two effects on the nervous system are possible, one on the spinal cord itself (myelopathy), and the other an effect on the spinal cord nerve roots (radiculopathy).

Myelopathy in cervical spondylosis.—Among the large number of adults who develop cervical spondylosis are a small number who

---

FIG. 52 (*see opposite*)

(*a*) Spinal canal, opened from behind by laminectomy, from a case of cervical spondylosis. The dura mater has been opened and the spinal cord (Fig. 52*b*) removed.

(*b*) Spinal cord, seen from its anterior aspect, and showing indentations caused by spondylotic protrusions.

(*c*) Transverse sections through C6 spinal cord segment of a case of cervical spondylosis. Note the indentations of the anterior aspect of the spinal cord, the leptomeningeal fibrosis and the intense vascular proliferation throughout the cord. Haematoxylin and Van Gieson ×8.

proceed to develop a spinal-cord syndrome. This is manifested clinically as a very mild and very slowly progressive quadriparesis made up of a spastic paraparesis together with, in a few cases, some lower motor neurone impairment in the arms. There may also be sensory changes and disturbance of bowel and bladder function.

The radiological changes are: loss of cervical lordosis, narrowing of intervertebral disc spaces, osteophytosis with encroachment on the intervertebral foramina or the spinal canal, sclerosis of the vertebral margins, and narrowing (anteroposteriorly) of the spinal canal. The cerebrospinal fluid is normal, but sometimes a manometric block can be shown if the neck is extended. Myelography shows posterior filling defects opposite a disc space, and the best views are obtained with the patient prone and the neck hyperextended.

The clinical course of these cases is that of slow progression over years and this can be halted by the simple expedient of limiting neck movements by some form of collar. Various surgical operations on the spinal deformity have their advocates, but the results are not encouraging and compare unfavourably with the success of simple neck immobilisation.

The pathology of this condition has not been demonstrated as conclusively as might at first sight appear, since in the majority of cases the diagnosis is not verified at necropsy. Reports with necropsy observations were published by Bedford et al. (1952), one case; Brain et al. (1952), six cases; Mair and Druckman (1953), four cases; Wilkinson (1960), 17 cases. In my own experience I have examined at necropsy twenty cases, whose diagnosis during life was cervical spondylosis. Of these only eight cases proved to have the syndrome we are discussing. The remainder had undiagnosed conditions such as multiple sclerosis, atherosclerotic vascular disease, and meningioma (one case). In five cases the cervical spondylosis was combined with a hyperextension injury to the cervical spine, a complication that has been reviewed elsewhere (Hughes and Brownell, 1963). My experience of the pathology of cervical spondylosis has been enlarged by cases found in a prospective necropsy series of 200 consecutive adult necropsies, and in this series 15 cases with myelopathy and six cases with radiculopathy due to cervical spondylosis were discovered.

The most conspicuous macroscopical features in the spinal canal are the posterior bulges associated with the affected intervertebral discs. These may be transverse bars extending across the whole transverse diameter of the spinal canal or they may be localised bulges either central or lateral. The lateral bulges may encroach on an intervertebral foramen and cause pressure on a nerve root. In the most severely affected spines there are large osteophytes affecting consecutive disc spaces and the bulges merge into a smooth encroachment on the spinal canal. These cases are often the worst, judged by the narrowing produced in the antero-posterior diameter of the canal. The spinal cord shows indentation (Fig. 52*b*) corresponding to the spondylotic protrusions (Fig. 52*a*); these are sometimes exaggerated by post-mortem moulding during fixation, but often their significance can be shown by localised histological changes. The meninges do not show, in my experience, any great changes. The dura may be thickened and adherent to a thickened periosteum, but there are rarely any adhesions between leptomeninges and dura.

The histological examination of the spinal cord (Fig. 52*c*) shows a varying degree of damage ranging from quite minor changes, the significance of which is difficult to assess. All the following changes should be observed in order to justify the pathological diagnosis of myelopathy caused by cervical spondylosis.

1. Posterior column long-tract degeneration. If this is present both at the levels C1 and T1 then the degeneration must be more evident at the upper level.
2. Lateral column long-tract degeneration. If this is present both at the levels C1 and T1 then the degeneration must be greater at the lower level.
3. White matter destruction, such as irregular areas of myelin pallor or necrosis.
4. Grey matter destruction, such as loss of neurones or ischaemic changes in the grey matter.

All cases with myelopathy show deformity due to indentation of the spinal cord by the spondylotic protrusions. The converse is not true since occasionally a markedly indented cord has no clinical or pathological evidence of myelopathy. The other change, which is very constant, is a widespread proliferation of small vessels which have a surrounding condensation of hyaline connective tissue.

TABLE I

Measurements on 200 cervical spines of consecutive adult necropsies

Macroscopical examination of cervical spine	Microscopical examination of spinal cord	No. of cases	Narrowest A-P diameter of cervical canal	Size of protrusions Vertical × transverse	No. of protrusions per case
Normal	Normal	93	14.3 mm (1.414)*		
Spondylosis	Normal	86	12.1 mm (1.483)*	7.3 × 14.1 mm	2.29
Spondylosis	Myelopathy	15	11.3 mm (1.678)*	8.3 × 15.4 mm	3.07
Spondylosis	Radiculopathy	6	11.7 mm (0.3316)*	7.0 × 13.7 mm	3.33

* Standard deviation.

The mechanism by which the spinal cord is damaged in cervical spondylosis remains unproven. In my own experience, the narrowing of the anteroposterior diameter of the spinal canal produced by the spondylotic protrusions has transcended in importance any other single finding. This impression was strengthened by a statistical analysis of the A–P diameters, measured intradurally, on 15 cases of myelopathy discovered in an examination of the cervical spine in 200 consecutive adult necropsies. Table I summarises some of the relevant measurements obtained. It will be seen that the cases with myelopathy had more spondylotic protrusions and that these were larger and narrowed the canal more than in the cases with cervical spondylosis but with microscopically normal spinal cords. The most important measurement is probably the narrowest A–P diameter of the cervical canal and the mean of these was 11.3 mm in the cases with myelopathy and 12.1 mm in the cases without spinal cord involvement. Similar findings were obtained in an analysis of the A–P diameters of the spinal cords.

Table II shows the mean of the ages and also the sex incidence of each group. As might be expected, the mean age of all the groups with spondylosis exceeds the mean age of the group without spondylosis. But also it can be seen that the group with

TABLE II

Mean Ages and Sex incidence of 200 cervical spines of consecutive adult necropsies

Macroscopical examination of cervical spine	Microscopical examination of spinal cord	No. of cases	Mean age	Sex	
				Male	Female
Normal	Normal	93	57.3	57 61.3%	36 38.7%
Spondylosis	Normal	86	69.6	46 53.5%	40 46.5%
Spondylosis	Myelopathy	15	72.0	13 86.7%	2 13.3%
Spondylosis	Radiculopathy	6	73.5	4 66.7%	2 33.3%

myelopathy (and that with radiculopathy) have a higher mean age than the groups without spinal cord involvement. The sex incidence shows a striking male prevalence, present even when corrected for the overall male excess of the whole population. This finding, in agreement with clinical observation, is probably of etiological significance and possibly reflects some occupational factor in the causation of the spinal cord pathology.

Whilst the evidence points to the importance of a narrow spinal canal, it is still not clear how the spinal cord is damaged. Mair and Druckman (1953) considered the damage to lie in the territory of the anterior spinal vessels, but occlusion of the anterior spinal artery is very rare in this condition (Hughes and Brownell, 1964) and gives a different clinical picture. It may be that the effect on these vessels is exerted by repeated frictional injury (Logue, 1957). Compression of the vertebral artery by osteophytes has been suggested (Sheehan et al., 1960; Hardin et al., 1960; Bauer et al., 1961) and appears, from these reports, to cause a syndrome of vertebrobasilar insufficiency provoked by neck movements. I could not demonstrate any occlusion or stenosis in my own cases but it is possible that during life the vertebral arteries were abnormally compressed during neck movements. Frykholm (1951) has emphasised the importance of root-sleeve fibrosis in fixing the spinal cord in the canal. Such immobility would also seem to be enforced by the moulding of the spinal cord around the spondylotic protrusions. Immobility of the spinal cord in the canal may predispose to damage during neck movements. It has been shown that the ligamentum flavum bulges anteriorly during neck extension and in this added compression to a spondylotic spinal canal may lie the hazard of neck movement (Taylor, 1953; Nugent, 1959; Reid, 1960; Stoltmann and Blackwood, 1964).

Adams and Logue (1971a, b, and c) have in a series of investigations resolved some of these doubtful points. In their first paper they report observations based on X-rays taken in flexion and extension of the head and neck in ten cadavers. The movement of the dura, roots and spinal cord in the cervical region was observed by the insertion of wire and pin markers. The extrathecal spinal roots were found to be fixed in the outer part of the intervertebral foramina but to move upwards and downwards with respect to the spinal canal. The dural sac was found to move, mainly by shifting, but partly by unfolding and stretching of that part subjected to traction. The movement of the spinal cord was the same as that of the dural sac except that in the upper cervical region the cord moved up less than the dura during flexion. Like Reid (1960) they found ascending extrathecal roots. These are known to be commoner with age and are probably explained by shortening of the spine due to disc degeneration whilst the dural sac remains a constant length.

In their second paper Adams and Logue (1971b) reported measurements on the range of movement and the structural appearance on X-rays in three groups of patients: a control group, a group with spondylotic myelopathy and a group with spondylotic radiculopathy. Cervical spines in the control group (with or without cervical spondylosis) differed from spines associated with radiculopathy or myelopathy in respect of the amount of kyphosis and lordosis developed in relation to the range of movement. They concluded that root or cord compression alone would not explain all cases of spondylotic radiculopathy and myelopathy. The effect of movement on the deformed spine is probably the key factor.

Their last paper reported results on 27 patients treated by posterior laminectomy (24 cases) or by anterior interbody fusion (three cases). Improvement was greatest in those patients who had the greatest limitation of neck movements after the operations. Relief of compression seemed of less importance than limitation of movement.

Radiculopathy in cervical spondylosis.—The spinal nerve roots are affected by spondylotic protrusions which occur either into the lateral part of the spinal canal or into the intervertebral foramen. The syndrome of brachialgia so caused is a common disability whose clinical aspects should be sought elsewhere (Logue, 1957).

The pathological findings in these cases are the bony and cartilaginous changes of spondylosis involving certain spinal nerve roots. Although these cases are common, reports of necropsies are rare and most of the large series, with morbid anatomical descriptions, refer to cases in which the roots have been inspected during an operation designed to relieve them of compression. My experience of necropsied cases is confined to six cases with radiculopathy and these were discovered, as has been described for myelopathy, in a prospective search of a series of 200 adult necropsies. It is likely that radiculopathy often accompanies myelopathy but then the microscopical features, at least in the spinal cord, are obscured. In a case in which the radiculopathy predominates the pattern of Wallerian degeneration in the posterior columns is very characteristic. The central fibres of one or more posterior columns are involved and the fibres concerned become more compact and more medially situated as one examines successively higher cervical cord segments. This pattern of fibre degeneration, also seen after posterior rhizotomy, is pathognomonic of a lesion of the posterior nerve roots.

The particular osteophytic changes leading to radiculopathy were studied by Payne and Spillane (1957) in serial sections of decalcified cervical spines. In my own cases the extent of the foraminal narrowing was examined radiologically. It is the uncovertebral osteophyte which, protruding into the intervertebral foramen, causes the foraminal narrowing. Payne and Spillane found the greatest effect of this compression exerted on the radicular nerve and the posterior root ganglion, whilst the anterior root was frequently spared.

RHEUMATOID ARTHRITIS

In the disease rheumatoid arthritis there is, within a generalised connective tissue inflammatory process, a characteristic polyarthritis with a predilection for the smaller joints of the body. The disease is three times as common in females as in males (compare ankylosing spondylitis) and tends to begin in young adult life. In some of the earliest accounts of rheumatoid arthritis (Garrod, 1890) the involvement of the cervical spine was described. Rheumatoid arthritis usually affects the spinal cord or its nerve roots by a dislocation in the cervical region. This dislocation is most commonly seen between the first and second cervical vertebrae and this *atlanto-axial dislocation* is somewhat different from dislocation below the second vertebra which is termed *subaxial* dislocation.

Atlanto-axial Dislocation

There are many clinical accounts of atlanto-axial dislocation in rheumatoid arthritis of which the following list is a short selection: Lourie and Stewart (1961), Margulies *et al.* (1955), Martel and Abell (1963). The review of Ball and Sharp (1971) includes a pathological description based on two necropsies

The condition is not uncommon in a busy neuropathological practice but good descriptions at necropsy are rare.

The spine itself is usually affected by severe osteoporosis and this change may, in addition to a general malleability of the skeleton, cause loosening of the various ligamentous attachments to bone. The main ligaments securing the atlas and axis to one another and to the skull are the transverse ligaments of the atlas (mooring the odontoid process to the atlas) and the two alar ligaments (attaching the odontoid process to the occipital condyles). The apical ligament attaches the apex of the odontoid to the anterior edge of the foramen magnum. The superior and inferior longitudinal bands attach the atlas to the occiput above and to the axis below. These two ligaments form, with the transverse ligament, the cruciform ligament of the atlas. There are also important capsular ligaments surrounding the atlanto-occipital joint and the atlanto-axial joint. All these ligaments may be weakened by a destructive inflammatory process similar to that described in the tendons of the hand in cases of rheumatoid arthritis. The intervertebral joints also are attacked by a chronic destructive arthritis which, together with the osteoporosis and the ligamentous weakening, causes serious loosening of the joints. The consequence is a bilateral dislocation usually of the atlanto-occipital joint with the atlas usually moving forward with respect to the axis. The dislocation may remain mobile or may become fixed by fibrosis or bony ankylosis.

The spinal cord is affected by pressure because the spinal canal is narrowed anteroposteriorly due to the kyphosis at the place of dislocation. Despite the deformity, the spinal cord degeneration frequently is minimal and the clinical picture is that of a spastic paraparesis or quadriparesis. The grey matter may be affected by ischaemia due to pressure on the anterior spinal artery. Root lesions may be demonstrable and are caused by the involvement of spinal nerve roots passing through distorted intervertebral foramina.

Subaxial Dislocation

Rheumatoid arthritis affects the spine due to involvement of the neurocentral and apophyseal joints in the chronic arthritis which causes bony destruction without the stabilising effect of osteophyte formation. In this particular, the rheumatoid neck differs

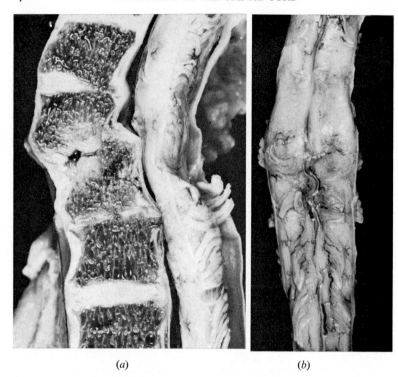

(a)   (b)

FIG. 53.—Rheumatoid arthritis with myelopathy.
   (a) Right half of a sagittally sawn specimen of cervical spine from C3 to C7. There is subluxation forward of the spine down to C4 with respect to the part from C5 downwards. Note the deformity produced in the spinal cord.
   (b) Anterior aspect of spinal cord showing compression at C4 spinal cord segment.

significantly from the condition cervical spondylosis. The neuro-central joints unite the lateral part of the vertebral bodies whilst the apophyseal joints join an inferior articular process above to a superior articular process below. The weakening of these joints by a destructive arthritis which also destroys bone and inter-vertebral disc causes a bilateral dislocation. The dislocation may be mobile but more often becomes relatively fixed by fibrosis or rigid by a bony ankylosis. In two cases I have examined at necropsy the dislocation was between C4 and C5 with forward luxation of the upper portion with respect to the lower portion (Fig. 53a). Consequently the upper and posterior part of the C5 body projected backwards into the spinal canal severely narrowing and distorting the lumen.

The spinal cord is affected by pressure with moulding of the cord around the deformity (Fig. 53b). The leptomeninges show marked fibrosis whilst the cord itself shows grey and white matter degeneration with evidence of ischaemia. Above the critical area there is upward Wallerian degeneration in the posterior columns whilst below there is corticospinal tract degeneration.

Ankylosing Spondylitis

This arthropathy, also called Marie-Strümpell spondylitis and Von Bechterew-Strümpell spondylitis, is a chronic progressive arthritis affecting mainly the sacro-iliac joints and the apophyseal joints of the spine, although the hip and shoulder joints are sometimes involved. The condition is much commoner in males but in both sexes has an interesting and important association with the HL-A tissue antigen system.

As in rheumatoid arthritis atlanto-axial dislocation can occur (Sharp and Purser, 1961). Also a cauda equina syndrome has been described (Matthews, 1968) in which arachnoid adhesions and numerous large arachnoid cysts have been found at necropsy. These cysts, which can sometimes be seen during life by myelography, appear to be a late sequel of a chronic arachnoiditis. It is of interest that the early descriptions of this disease by Von Bechterew mentioned this involvement of the spinal meninges.

REFERENCES

DEVELOPMENTAL ABNORMALITIES OF THE SPINAL CANAL

BACHS, A., BARRAQUER-BORDAS, L., BARRAQUER-FERRÉ, L., CANADELL, J. M. and MODOLELL, A. (1955). Delayed myelopathy following atlanto-axial dislocation by separated odontoid process. *Brain*, **78**, 537–552.

BHARUCHA, E. P. and DASTUR, H. M. (1964). Craniovertebral anomalies. *Brain*, **87**, 469–480.

BULL, J. W. B., NIXON, W. L. B. and PRATT, R. T. C. (1955). The radiological criteria and familial occurrence of primary basilar impression. *Brain*, **78**, 229–247.

DASTUR, D. K., WADIA, N. H., DESAI, A. D. and SINH, G. (1965). Medullospinal compression due to atlanto-axial dislocation and sudden haematomyelia during decompression. *Brain*, **88**, 897–924.

DONATH, J. and VOGL, A. (1925). Chrondrodystrophic dwarfs. *Wien Arch. inn. Med.*, **10**, 1–44.

DUVOISIN, R. C. and YAHR, M. D. (1962). Compressive spinal cord and root syndromes in achondroplastic dwarfs. *Neurology* (*Minneap.*), **12**, 202–207.

EPSTEIN, J. A. and MALIS, L. I. (1955). Compression of spinal cord and cauda equina in achondroplastic dwarfs. *Neurology* (*Minneap.*), **5**, 875–881.

FREUND, E. (1933). Spastic paraplegia in achondroplasia. *Arch. Surg.*, **27**, 859–867.

MCRAE, D. L. (1953). Bony abnormalities in the region of the foramen magnum: correlation of the anatomic and neurologic findings. *Acta radiol.* (*Stockh.*), **40**, 335–354.

SPILLANE, J. D. (1952). Three cases of achondroplasia with neurological complications. *J. Neurol. Neurosurg. Psychiat.*, **15**, 246–252.

SPILLANE, J. D., PALLIS, C. and JONES, A. M. (1957). Developmental abnormalities in the region of the foramen magnum. *Brain*, **80**, 11–48.

VOGL, A. and OSBORNE, R. L. (1949). Lesions of spinal cord (transverse myelopathy) in achondroplasia. *Arch. Neurol. Psychiat.* (*Chic.*), **61**, 644–662.

TOXIC AND METABOLIC DISORDERS OF THE SPINE

BRENNER, H. (1962). Paraplegie infolge isoliertem Morbus Paget der Brustwirbelsäule. *Zbl. Neurochir.*, **23**, 103–109.

CULLEN, D. R. and PEARCE, J. M. S. (1964). Spinal cord compression in pseudohypoparathyroidism. *J. Neurol. Neurosurg. Psychiat.*, **27**, 459–462.

DUGGER, G. S. and VANDIVER, R. W. (1966). Spinal cord compression caused by vitamin-D-resistant rickets. *J. Neurosurg.*, **25**, 300–303.

ELKINGTON, J. ST. C. (1939). Paget's disease with paraplegia. *Proc. roy. Soc. Med.*, **32**, 1420–1421.

KENNEDY, P., SWASH, M. and DEAN, M. F. (1973). Cervical cord compression in mucopolysaccharidosis. *Develop. Med. Child. Neurol.*, **15**, 194–199.

RAYNOR, R. B. (1962). Spinal-cord compression secondary to Gaucher's disease. Case report. *J. Neurosurg.*, **19**, 902–905.

SHORTT, H. E., MCROBERT, G. R., BARNARD, T. W. and NAYAR, A. S. M. (1937). Endemic fluorosis in the Madras Presidency. *Ind. J. med. Res.*, **25**, 553–554, 568.

SIDDIQUI, A. H. (1955). Fluorosis in Nalgonda district, Hyderabad-Deccan. *Brit. med. J.*, **2**, 1408–1413.

SINGH, A., JOLLY, S. S. and BANSAL, B. C. (1961). Skeletal fluorosis and its neurological complications. *Lancet*, **1**, 197–200.

SINGH, A., JOLLY, S. S., BANSAL, B. C. and MATHUR, C. C. (1963). Endemic fluorosis. Epidemiological, clinical, and biochemical study of chronic fluorine intoxication in Panjab (India). *Medicine* (*Baltimore*), **42**, 229–246.

TENG, P., GROSS, S. W. and NEWMAN, C. M. (1951). Compression of spinal cord by osteitis deformans (Paget's disease), giant-cell tumour and polyostotic fibrous dysplasia (Albright's syndrome) of vertebrae. *J. Neurosurg.*, **8**, 482–493.

TEOTIA, M., TEOTIA, S. P. S. and KUNWAR, K. B. (1971). Endemic skeletal fluorosis. *Arch. Dis. Childh.*, **46**, 686–691.

TURNER, J. W. A. (1940). The spinal complication of Paget's disease (osteitis deformans). *Brain*, **63**, 321–349.

WYLLIE, W. G. (1923). The occurrence in osteitis deformans of lesions of the central nervous system with a report of four cases. *Brain*, **46**, 336–351.

DEGENERATIVE DISEASES OF THE SPINE

ADAMS, C. B. T. and LOGUE, V. (1971*a*). Studies in cervical spondylotic myelopathy. I. *Brain*, **94**, 557–568.

ADAMS, C. B. T. and LOGUE, V. (1971*b*). Studies in cervical spondylotic myelopathy. II. *Brain*, **94**, 569–586.

ADAMS, C. B. T. and LOGUE, V. (1971*c*). Studies in cervical spondylotic myelopathy. III. *Brain*, **94**, 587–594.

BALL, J. and SHARP, J. (1971). Rheumatoid arthritis of the cervical spine. In *Modern Trends in Rheumatology.* Ed. by A. G. S. Hill. London: Butterworths.

BAUER, R., SHEEHAN, S. and MEYER, J. S. (1961). Arteriographic study of cerebrovascular disease. *Arch. Neurol. (Chic.)*, **4**, 119–131.

BEDFORD, P. D., BOSANQUET, F. D. and RUSSELL, W. R. (1952). Degeneration of cervical cord associated with cervical spondylosis. *Lancet*, **2**, 55–59.

BRAIN, W. R., NORTHFIELD, D. and WILKINSON, MARCIA (1952). The neurological manifestations of cervical spondylosis. *Brain*, **75**, 187–225.

CLARKE, E. and ROBINSON, D. K. (1956). Cervical myelopathy: a complication of cervical spondylosis. *Brain*, **79**, 483–510.

FRYKHOLM, R. (1951). Cervical nerve root compression resulting from disc degeneration and root-sleeve fibrosis. A clinical investigation. *Acta chir. scand.*, Suppl. 160.

GARROD, A. E. (1890). *A Treatise on Rheumatism and Rheumatoid Arthritis.* London: Griffin.

GOLDTHWAIT, J. E. (1911). The lumbo-sacral articulation; an explanation of many cases of "lumbago", "sciatica" and paraplegia. *Boston med. surg. J.*, **164**, 365–372.

HARDIN, C. A., WILLIAMSON, W. D. and STEEGMAN, T. A. (1960). Vertebral artery insufficiency produced by cervical osteoarthritic spurs. *Neurology (Minneap.)*, **10**, 855–858.

HUGHES, J. T. and BROWNELL, B. (1963). Spinal-cord damage from hyperextension injury in cervical spondylosis. *Lancet.* **1**, 678–690.

182   PATHOLOGY OF THE SPINAL CORD

HUGHES, J. T. and BROWNELL, B. (1964). Cervical spondylosis complicated by anterior spinal artery thrombosis. *Neurology (Minneap.)*, **14**, 1073–1077.

KOCHER, T. (1896). Die Verletzungen der Wirbelsäule zugleich als Beitrag zur Physiologie des menschlichen Rückenmarks. *Mitt. Grenzgeb. Med. Chir.*, **1**, 415–480.

LOGUE, V. (1957). Cervical spondylosis. In *Modern Trends in Neurology*, 2nd series. Ed. by D. Williams. London: Butterworth.

LOURIE, H. and STEWART, W. A. (1961). Spontaneous atlanto-axial dislocation; a complication of rheumatoid disease. *New Engl. J. Med.*, **265**, 677–681.

LUSCHKA, H. VON (1858). *Die Halbgelenke des menschlichen Körpers.* Berlin: Reimer.

MAIR, W. G. P. and DRUCKMAN, R. (1953). The pathology of spinal cord lesions and their relation to the clinical features in protrusions of cervical intervertebral discs. *Brain*, **76**, 70–91.

MARGULIES, M. E., KATZ, I. and ROSENBERG, M. (1955). Spontaneous dislocation of the atlanto-axial joint in rheumatoid spondylitis: recovery from quadriplegia following surgical decompression. *Neurology (Minneap.)*, **5**, 290–294.

MARTEL, W. and ABELL, M. R. (1963). Fatal atlanto-axial luxation in rheumatoid arthritis. *Arthr. and Rheum.*, **6**, 224–231.

MATTHEWS, W. B. (1968). The neurological complications of ankylosing spondylitis. *J. neurol. Sci.*, **6**, 561–573.

MIDDLETON, G. S. and TEACHER, J. H. (1911). Injury of the spinal cord due to rupture of an intervertebral disc during muscular effort. *Glasg. med. J.*, **76**, 1–6.

MIXTER, W. J. (1951). Rupture of the intervertebral disc. In *Modern Trends in Neurology*, 1st series. Ed. by A. Feiling. London: Butterworth.

NACHEMSON, A. and MORRIS, J. (1963). Lumbar discometry; lumbar intradiscal pressure measurements *in vivo*. *Lancet*, **1**, 1140–1142.

NUGENT, G. R. (1959). Clinicopathologic correlations in cervical spondylosis. *Neurology (Minneap.)*, **9**, 273–281.

PAYNE, E. E. and SPILLANE, J. D. (1957). The cervical spine. An anatomicopathological study of 70 specimens with particular reference to the problem of cervical spondylosis. *Brain*, **80**, 571–596.

REID, J. D. (1960). Effects of flexion-extension movements of the head and spine upon the spinal cord and nerve roots. *J. Neurol. Neurosurg. Psychiat.*, **23**, 214–221.

SANDLER, B. (1961). Cervical spondylosis as a cause of spinal cord pathology. *Arch. phys. Med.*, **42**, 650–660.

SCHMORL, G. and JUNGHANS, H. (1959). *The Human Spine in Health and Disease.* 1st American edit. translated and edited by S. P. Wilk. New York: Grune and Stratton.

SHARP, J. and PURSER, D. W. (1961). Spontaneous atlanto-axial dislocation in ankylosing spondylitis and rheumatoid arthritis. *Ann. rheum. Dis.*, **20**, 47–77.

SHEEHAN, S., BAUER, R. B. and MEYER, J. S. (1960). Vertebral artery compression in cervical spondylosis. *Neurology (Minneap.)*, **10**, 968–986.

STOLTMANN, H. F. and BLACKWOOD, W. (1964). The role of the ligamenta flava in the pathogenesis of myelopathy in cervical spondylosis. *Brain*, **87**, 45–50.

TAYLOR, A. R. (1953). Mechanism and treatment of spinal-cord disorders associated with cervical spondylosis. *Lancet*, **1**, 717–720.

WILKINSON, M. (1960). The morbid anatomy of cervical spondylosis and myelopathy. *Brain*, **83**, 589–617.

CHAPTER VIII

TOXIC AND DEFICIENCY DISEASES

In the group of toxic and deficiency diseases only subacute combined degeneration of the cord accounts for an important number of cases, at least in the developed countries of the world. Nevertheless it is justified to describe the toxic and nutritional states that can affect the spinal cord since these diseases can be prevented. In some parts of the world nutritional deficiency states are so prevalent as to constitute the chief disease group, and occasionally a toxic disease can suddenly appear in epidemic proportions as happened in the outbreak in Morocco of tri-orthocresyl phosphate poisoning in 1959.

TOXIC DISEASES

Apart from chemical poisons, toxic states can arise from radio-therapy, electric shock and lightning stroke. X-ray myelopathy is an important hazard in the therapy of malignant tumours and has attracted considerable interest. The effects of electrocution and lightning stroke have received little attention but in both a spinal cord syndrome can result (Langworthy, 1932; Alexander, 1938). Apart from these noxious mechanisms, toxic agents enter the body by being ingested, inhaled or parenterally injected. Pentschew (1958, 1971) reviews the pathology of the various intoxications which affect the nervous system. In the case of the spinal cord a distinct group of disorders occurs from toxins reaching the spinal subarachnoid space and so directly damaging the spinal cord.

Radiation Myelopathy

In 1945 Stevenson and Eckhardt reported the case of a man of 43 years who, two years after receiving radiation in a dosage of 6,000–8,000 rad for a lymphoepithelioma of the nasopharynx, developed a spinal cord syndrome, which proved at autopsy to be caused by the radiation. Ahlbom (1941) had previously described the clinical syndrome following the radiotherapy of hypopharyngeal cancer. Subsequently the pathological changes were described in other necropsied cases by Boden (1948), Malamud et al. (1954)

and Itabashi *et al.* (1957). Many cases must escape detection and Boden (1948, 1950) in a search among 161 patients with irradiation of regions near the cervical spinal cord found 13 cases of radiation myelopathy. Further cases have been reported by, among others, Pallis *et al.* (1961), Dynes and Smedal (1960), Jellinger and Sturm (1971), Henry *et al.* (1971), Burns *et al.* (1971) and Palmer (1972). Most of the cases quoted have been caused by irradiation to the cervical cord but many of those of Dynes and Smedal affected the upper thoracic region which they consider, when exposed to high-dosage radiation, to be more vulnerable than other parts of the spinal cord.

Clinical features.—The onset of the myelopathy is usually about a year after the radiotherapy, but latent periods of as little as one month and as long as 70 months have been reported. Having begun, the process is steadily progressive often to a fatal outcome in a few months. The first symptoms are usually dysaesthesiae of the limbs which become weak and, in the cervical cases, a flaccid areflexic paralysis of the arms is accompanied by a spastic paraparesis. Paralysis of bladder and bowel is common and is a bad prognostic sign. Myelography has been normal and the only change in the spinal fluid has been a slight elevation of the protein level. There is no known treatment but occasionally the pace of deterioration slackens and survival for several years is possible. Correct diagnosis is important as otherwise more irradiation may be given in the hope of treating an intramedullary metastasis of the original tumour.

Pathological features.—All the case reports with detailed necropsy observations describe areas of necrosis and regions of lesser damage having the appearance in the white matter of spongy degeneration, whilst the neurones are described as showing vacuolation and other degenerative changes. In the case of Itabashi *et al.*, a round area of necrosis involved the left side of the cord, which elsewhere was more diffusely damaged. Wallerian degeneration was commonly present in these cases and in extent was appropriate to the position of the areas of necrosis. The leptomeninges sometimes showed fibrous thickening. Most of the observers have emphasised vascular changes which are thought to explain the necrosis. There are many new vessels in the affected regions, both capillaries and arterioles. The walls of the capillaries are thickened with hyaline change and the arterioles showed mural hypertrophy with a lumen smaller than normal. The veins often appear dilated and congested. This vascular reaction, to which the necrosis may be secondary, is known to be a consequence of radiotherapy, but why it should occur only in a proportion of cases and after a variable, usually long, interval is a mystery.

This "vascular" explanation of radiation myelopathy has not gone unchallenged and Burns *et al.* (1972) favour a direct effect on the neural elements by the radiation. Other workers (quoted by Palmer, 1972) suggest an immunological mechanism for the delayed effects of radiation on the nervous system.

Barbotage

Aspiration and reinjection (barbotage) of cerebrospinal fluid, both in experimental animals (Bunge and Settlage, 1957) and in human cases (Friede and Roessmann, 1969) results in the destruction of myelinated fibres in a thin marginal layer at the surface of the spinal cord, brain stem and optic nerves. The effect is capricious, being inconstant in appearance and variable in location. The affected surface areas tend to be near the site of aspiration and this and other features suggest a pressure effect. The effect on myelin has been used frequently as an experimental model of myelin destruction and also in human patients for pain relief (Lloyd *et al.*, 1972). The appearance in the spinal cord is very striking and the small number of human cases so far reported suggests that CSF manipulation in human patients rarely produces this florid myelin destruction.

Toxic Myelopathy from Chemical Poisons

Many inorganic poisons affect the nervous system but any damage to the spinal cord is usually overshadowed by the effect on the brain. This is so in heavy-metal poisoning, the chief examples of which are copper, mercury and lead. Lead may cause a polyneuropathy but then its effect on the spinal cord is a secondary one. One report of lead causing a myelopathy will be described. Organic poisons, both industrial and pharmaceutical, are very much commoner and the list of compounds affecting the nervous system is very long. Arsphenamine medication has occasionally caused myelopathy (Glaser, 1934; Blankenhorn and Wolff, 1948) but such cases must now be very rare. More important is the occasional toxicity of some antimalarial drugs such as pamaquin, since suppressive therapy for malaria is widespread in large areas of the world. Pamaquin and related drugs have been found toxic to monkeys and a fatal human case was described by Löken and Haymaker (1949). Partial necrosis of brain stem and spinal cord is described both in monkeys and in the human case.

Lead Myelopathy

Boehme (1971) described the case of a 66-year-old man, a foundry worker, who developed a myelopathy in which lead salts were found in the spinal cord as deposits in the grey and white matter, around the blood vessels, and as subpial plaque-like deposits. The material was analysed by X-ray crystallography and laser microprobe spectometry and was found to consist of hydrocerussite (lead carbonate and lead hydroxide).

Ortho-cresyl Phosphate Poisoning

Triorthocresyl phosphate is the most notorious of these compounds all of which are neurotoxic, apparently due to selective enzymatic poisoning of certain neurones (Cavanagh, 1954). There are many reports of sporadic cases resulting from accidental ingestion, but very large numbers of cases occurred in the U.S.A. during prohibition in 1930 from drinking "Jamaica ginger" (Smith and Lillie, 1931). A large outbreak occurred in Meknes in Morocco due to the contamination of cooking oil by synthetic lubricating oil containing orthocresyl phosphate (Smith and Spalding, 1959).

Clinical course.—The clinical picture in these epidemics was that of an acute polyneuropathy developing over a period of weeks and causing widespread but mainly distal paralysis first of the lower limbs and later the hands. Spinal cord involvement either accompanied or followed the peripheral neuropathy and added an upper motor neurone lesion to the paralysis.

Pathological changes in the spinal cord.—Despite the severity of the paralysis, in every outbreak the mortality of the condition has been low and consequently there have been few necropsies. Reports known to the author are those of Vonderahe (1931), Smith and Lillie (1931), Kidd and Langworthy (1933) and Aring (1942); the last named report deals with the late pathological findings. The spinal cords showed leptomeningeal thickening. White matter degeneration was always present, of variable distribution but always involving the lateral corticospinal tracts. The changes were much more marked in the lower cord than in the upper segments. The neuronal changes were less striking, there was a reduction of anterior horn cells and those remaining were sometimes pyknotic and lacked Nissl substance.

Transverse Myelitis Due to Opium Derivatives

Richter and Rosenberg (1968) published a report on four negro heroin addicts who developed transverse myelitis following intravenous heroin. These authors in an *addendum* mention two further cases and a similar case was described by Schein *et al.* (1971) in a white male who had injected himself with intravenous opium. The clinical history was similar in all these seven cases cited above. A syndrome of acute paraplegia affecting the thoracic region of the spinal cord developed following the intravenous injection of heroin or opium.

A necropsy was performed in case four of Richter and Rosenberg. The immediate cause of death was pulmonary embolism. The spinal cord was affected by a large area of softening extending from T9 to T11 spinal cord segments. At T10 a transverse section showed a large necrotic area involving all the grey matter and the adjacent white matter of the posterior columns, and this necrotic area was filled by lipid-laden phagocytes. No major arterial obstruction was found but the histological examination appears to have been limited to one spinal cord segment. Further pathological studies on cases of this nature are required. The circumstances of drug addiction, particularly when intravenous drugs are taken favour both sepsis and thrombo-embolism. These factors require exclusion before a direct toxic effect of opiates on the spinal cord is accepted.

Lathyrism

Lathyrism (Wilcocks and Manson-Bahr, 1972) is a disease endemic in Ethiopia, Algeria and India in districts where vetches such as *Lathyrus sativas* are consumed as food. The clinical syndrome is that of an acute ataxic spastic paraplegia and the pathology is that of degeneration of the corticospinal tracts in the spinal cord. There is an account of two necropsies in the paper by Dastur (1962).

Toxic Myelitis Following Aortography

This is a special example of neurotoxicity for the toxic agent is injected directly into the spinal cord arterial supply. Aortography, first described by dos Santos *et al.* (1929), is now a regular diagnostic aid in diseases of the aorta, major arteries, and some of the abdominal viscera. A variety of toxic effects have been described but of special importance is the occasional complication of paraplegia. The contrast media used include several iodine compounds but sodium acetrizoate has been responsible for a large number of the cases. It is probable that all iodine contrast media are to some extent injurious to the spinal cord, and their concentration in the spinal cord is perhaps the most important factor. The supine position of the patient is known to be hazardous, for then the heavy medium enters more readily the lumbar spinal arteries. The occurrence of this complication was traced by Killen and Foster (1960) who found 43 cases including those they reviewed in the world literature. The necropsy findings in a case of this complication were reported (Hughes and Brownell, 1965) and compared with four other published accounts. Cases have also been reported by Howieson and Megison (1968) and by Lyon (1971). There are several accounts of the experimental findings of contrast medium injury to the spinal cord of which that of Margolis et al. (1956) is recommended. In many subsequent experimental studies Margolis (see Margolis, 1970 for references) has demonstrated the great importance of the vascular bed into which the toxic agent is injected.

In human cases examined at necropsy the evidence favours a direct toxic action of the contrast medium on the spinal cord. The site and extent of the damage depend on the amount of the medium entering the spinal cord via the lumbar spinal arteries; the amount of damage varies from total necrosis to barely detectable loss of a few nerve fibres and neurone cell bodies. The histological appearance of the spinal cord in the acute stages is that of a toxic myelitis with destruction of white and grey matter alike. The destroyed tissue is then gradually removed and a case seen at a later stage shows atrophy of the part of the spinal cord affected.

Myelopathy Associated with Cirrhosis of the Liver

There are some 28 case reports in which paraplegia has developed in association with cirrhosis of the liver. The literature was reviewed by Pant et al. (1968), who added two other case reports. Subsequently Bechar et al. (1970) have recorded three further cases.

In most of the reported cases the paraplegia has developed after a portacaval anastomosis but sometimes no such surgical procedures have been performed but an extensive portacaval anastomosis has developed spontaneously. All the cases have severe liver failure and episodes of hepatic encephalopathy were a feature. The paraplegia is of gradual onset and insidious progression to a symmetrical spastic upper motor neurone paralysis. In the legs the tendon reflexes are exaggerated and the plantar responses were extensor. In one case some posterior column loss was present, otherwise sensation has been normal. A feature of the paraplegia has been its resistance to all the therapeutic measures employed.

Necropsy examinations have now been reported in several of the cases. The brain usually shows pathological evidence of hepatic encephalopathy with increase in size and in the numbers of astrocytes. There are degenerative changes in the corticospinal motor system with tract degeneration and reduction in the number of Betz cells. The spinal cords always show corticospinal tract degeneration and often posterior column degeneration. Some studies have suggested that the lesion in the spinal cord is one of demyelination but confirmation of this is required.

Further work is required to elucidate this interesting myelopathy whose cause is unknown. Its resistance to treatment suggests that nutritional deficiency, in particular avitaminosis B, is not the primary cause. It is known that portacaval shunt operations cause intoxication by nitrogenous metabolites which bypass the liver, and these toxic agents may cause the myelopathy.

Toxic Agents in the Subarachnoid Space

Alcohol and phenol have been used by injection into the subarachnoid space to relieve chronic pain or spasticity. In 1930 Dogliotti (Hay *et al.*, 1959) injected alcohol in this way to relieve pain, and Maher (1955) similarly used phenol. The position of the patient differs since alcohol being hypobaric rises in the spinal theca and so the patient is placed in a head-down position. Phenol is used mixed with radio-opaque medium and the resultant mixture, being hyperbaric, falls in the theca; so with phenol the patient must be erect for the desired effect. It is probable that the cases that rarely occur after spinal anaesthesia have a similar pathology due to accidental contamination by phenolic or other antiseptics (Hurst, 1955; Tsukagoshi *et al.*, 1970).

Berry and Olszewski (1963) have described the pathological features of intrathecal phenol in man; my own observations are in keeping with their findings. In the manner in which these agents are used in man they cause primarily a toxic radiculitis of the cauda equina. The affected nerve roots show damage to the outer nerve fibres and in a transverse section this affected peripheral zone is clearly defined from the inner preserved zone. The effects of this radiculopathy on the spinal cord are seen chiefly as ascending Wallerian degeneration in the posterior white columns and chromatolytic cells in the anterior grey horn.

Efocaine, a mixture of procaine, butyl amino benzoate, propylene, and propylene glycol, was formerly used by paravertebral injection as an anaesthetic blocking agent. Plum (1955) mentions eleven cases of transverse myelopathy caused by efocaine used in this manner, the likely explanation being the leakage of the drug into the subarachnoid space.

Penicillin, when used intrathecally in high concentration, must be considered a substance toxic to the spinal cord (Sweet et al., 1945). In 1944, when only impure preparations of penicillin were available, reactions to its intrathecal use occurred, but the modern purified product can be used in much greater concentration without mishap (Florey, 1952). It is possible that some cases have arisen from contamination of the drug or from added preservatives. Radiculomyelopathy has followed the intrathecal use of methylene blue (Schultz and Schwarz, 1970) and of fluorescien (Mahaley and Odom, 1966).

Adhesive Spinal Arachnoiditis

In all probability this condition is not a single pathological entity but the result of differing toxic processes, some of which remain unidentified. The etiological factors which have been suggested are trauma, spinal anaesthetics, myelography, subarachnoid haemorrhage and low-grade bacterial or viral infections. The subject has attracted much attention and the following papers are only a selection of the large literature on the subject: Kulowski and Scott (1934), Elkington (1936), Nelson (1943), French (1947), Nielsen (1952), Winkelman et al. (1953), Weiss et al. (1962), and Rétif et al. (1964). A great deal of experience of this and allied conditions is contained in the papers of Wadia and Dastur (1969) and Dastur and Wadia (1969).

Clinical features.—In such a heterogeneous group of conditions the clinical course is often diverse. The general pattern is a slowly progressive paraparesis combined with disturbances of sensation and of bladder and bowel function. The progress of the disability may be arrested or actual remission may occur; a change usually attributed to an improvement of the fluid dynamics of the spinal canal. A spinal block with Froin's syndrome is frequent and sometimes the greater part of the subarachnoid space is obliterated. The clinical course may simulate spinal cord tumour or syringomyelia. Exploratory laminectomy is usually performed for diagnosis and to exclude a remediable lesion. Some cases have been improved by removal of part or all of the thickened membrane.

Pathological findings.—The bulk of the reports describe a low-grade non-specific inflammatory reaction of the leptomeninges which in the later stages of the disease are thickened by acellular and avascular connective tissue. The abnormal findings may be widespread and circumscribed and in the localised forms there may be loculation of spinal fluid. Some of the large arachnoid cysts may arise in this way but others (Fig. 54), the proportion cannot be stated, are said to be developmental in origin. The spinal cord is often damaged by the leptomeningeal thickening and cavitation has been described. Some of the effects are due to pressure but a vascular disturbance caused by the involvement of small arteries in the leptomeningeal thickening is also likely.

DEFICIENCY DISEASES

The principal deficiency diseases affecting the spinal cord are caused by lack of vitamins of the B group. This group of vitamins is known to be complex not only in its component factors but in the diverse nutritional epidemics that may occur. Mixed deficiencies are common and the human disease frequently differs markedly from the experimental deficiency disease. Changes in the spinal cord have been reported in beri-beri, due to thiamin deficiency and in pellagra, due to lack of nicotinic acid. However in both these deficiencies changes in brain and peripheral nerve predominate. Having no personal experience, I refer the reader to the reviews of Pentschew (1958) and Meyer (1963). In the following deficiency disease due to avitaminosis B_{12} the spinal cord is predominantly involved.

Subacute Combined Degeneration of the Cord

This important disease was given its name by Russell *et al.* (1900), in an important paper, although antedated by less complete accounts. It was at that time recognised as a distinct clinical entity, usually but not invariably associated with anaemia. This association was clarified when the nature of pernicious anaemia was understood. With scarcely any exceptions the disease is associated with pernicious anaemia; the neurological disease may occur when the anaemia is subclinical or it may precede the development of

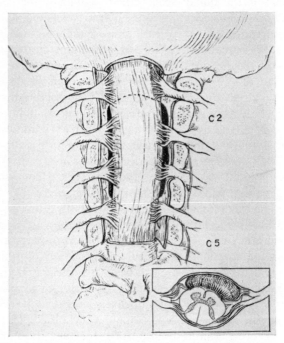

FIG. 54. Drawing of operative findings in a case of arachnoidal cyst in the cervical region.

the blood condition. For a full review of the literature the reader is referred to Erbslöh (1958). An excellent neuropathological account is that of Pant *et al.* (1968).

Clinical course.—The name of this condition may be cumbersome but it exactly states the clinical presentation. In the course of a few weeks or months the patient develops spastic weakness combined with ataxia and anaesthesia. The disability begins usually in the lower limbs but later also involves the trunk and arms. Sometimes the posterior column symptomatology and rarely the lateral column features predominate giving atypical clinical variants. Mental disorder is common in severe cases but there is no constant pattern. There may be peripheral nerve lesions and optic atrophy occurs. Without treatment the disease progresses rapidly but is arrested by liver therapy or by injections of vitamin B_{12} (cyanocobalamin); provided therapy with these drugs is regularly maintained, relapse does not occur.

Pathology in the spinal cord.—Macroscopically the spinal cord is normal or slightly swollen and on transverse slicing the long-tract degeneration in the white columns may be evident to the naked eye. Microscopically (Fig. 55a, b) the grey matter is scarcely affected and the changes in the white matter are best seen in a myelin stain of the Weigert type. The amount of degeneration found varies in each case and may be a few discrete lesions or a severe effect of almost the whole white matter, that remaining being usually a fringe around the grey matter. In addition to the inconstant amount of degeneration, the distribution is also variable. Erbslöh (1958) described a posterior column or tabetic type and a generalised type, in addition to the more usual combined type. In typical cases the thoracic region is the severest and earliest involved. The earliest lesions are in one or both posterior columns centrally, and in the lateral columns where they are peripherally situated. In late cases Wallerian degeneration imparts a spurious appearance of specific anatomical degeneration of fibre tracts. In the early cases and in atypical cases it is clear that the lesions are spherical or ovoid zones of degeneration, widespread, but with areas of predilection. This appearance is called in the German medical literature *Luckenfelder*, "fields of holes". The detailed histology of these lesions is important for they differ in certain respects from the plaques of multiple sclerosis. The earliest sign is a swelling of the myelin tubes, but axon degeneration accompanies the myelin change and the dissociated loss of the demyelinated plaque cannot be demonstrated. Sudan stains now show fat globules, some in lipid phagocytes. The spongy state has now developed, the strands of the sponge being astrocytes and their processes. There is no great proliferation of astrocytes as in the multiple sclerosis plaque, which is very different in its dense gliosis from the spongy state of the disease under discussion. With the progression of the disease a good deal of Wallerian degeneration adds to the picture as seen in transverse sections. The posterior columns and corticospinal tracts are usually the best outlined, but the spinocerebellar tracts are also degenerated; probably all

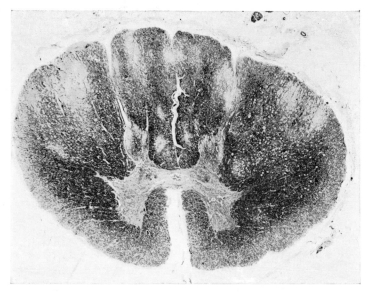

FIG. 55a.—Transverse section stained for myelin, at T5 segmental level, of an early case of subacute combined degeneration of the cord. Weil ×11.

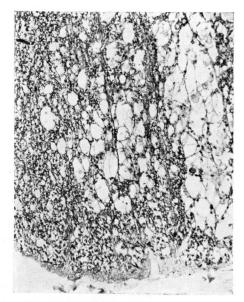

FIG. 55b.—Photomicrograph showing, at higher magnification, the spongy degeneration in the lateral columns of the case seen in Fig. 55a. Weil ×72.

long-fibre tracts eventually become affected. Due to the predominant involvement of the thoracic region the tract degeneration is less evident at the cephalic and caudal ends of the spinal cord.

Changes outside the spinal cord.—Similar lesions to those found in the spinal cord have been described in the cerebrum, brain stem, optic nerves and peripheral nerves. The other features are those of pernicious anaemia. The stomach mucosa is atrophic and the haemopoietic system is disordered by megaloblastic maturation of the erythrocytes and defective formation of white cells and platelets. The anaemia may be subclinical but more often a considerable diminution in haemoglobin adds the effects of a chronic and severe anaemia to the clinical and pathological picture.

Nutritional Myelopathy

One beneficial consequence of World War II was the careful study in considerable detail of the clinical course and sometimes of the pathology of the various nutritional syndromes affecting the central and peripheral nervous systems. Brain (1947), Denny-Brown (1947) and Spillane (1947) all had considerable experience of these syndromes in returning prisoners of war and the monograph of Spillane is highly recommended. All these three authors recognised a syndrome of spastic paraplegia which was quite distinct from the more common nutritional neuropathy and encephalopathy. Spillane saw seven cases of this syndrome, six from Changi camp and a seventh from a P.O.W. camp in Thailand. A recent paper on this condition is that of Grieve *et al.* (1967) who reported on a series of 61 cases of nutritional myelopathy occurring in the Bantu on the Witwatersrand. These cases came from people living on a very low dietary intake of vitamins, protein, and fat, the main constituent of their diet being maize porridge. Pellagra was present in the cases with glossitis, skin pigmentation, desquamation and diarrhoea.

The myelopathy is relatively slow in development but relentlessly progressive. The first physical signs are an increase in all the tendon reflexes. At a later stage there is a spastic paraparesis with lesser changes in the upper limbs. The final stage is a spastic paraplegia or quadriplegia with paralysis of bladder and of bowel. Sensory changes are rare. Mental abnormalities are common, but improve on treatment which has no effect on the myelopathy. In the seven cases seen by Spillane the syndrome began some four to six months after capture, had reached a maximum deficit in six weeks and was static, despite treatment, three years later.

Two necropsies were obtained in the series of Grieve *et al.* (1967). In both cases bilateral corticospinal tract degeneration was present and in one case there was also posterior column degeneration. More pathological data are required on further cases of this spastic paraplegia. There appears to be a general effect on the whole central nervous system with a preferential attack on the upper motor neurones. The condition must be carefully distinguished clinically and pathologically from lathyrism described earlier and from Jamaican (tropical) myeloneuropathy, now to be described.

Jamaican (Tropical) Myeloneuropathy

In the island of Jamaica for over a century a distinctive but complicated chronic neurological disease has been recognised. The condition is not confined to Jamaica but occurs throughout the West Indies and in West Indian immigrants into Britain and the United States. Some of the reports on the clinical and pathological features are reviewed by Robertson and Cruickshank (1972).

The syndrome consists of a mixture in varying proportions of spastic paraplegia, ataxia, and degeneration of the optic and auditory nerves. Clinically the cases divide into two types, spastic and ataxic. The ataxic type is uncommon and appears in a setting of severe malnutrition but without features suggesting a particular avitaminosis. No autopsy reports of this ataxia type have been described.

Spastic type.—This is the common form of the disease in Jamaica where it occurs in middle-aged negroes of either sex but without clear evidence of severe malnutrition. The disease begins with a spastic upper motor neurone weakness and (figures from Robertson and Cruickshank, 1972) is associated in 50 per cent of cases with ataxia, in 15 per cent of cases with optic atrophy, and in 7 per cent of cases with nerve deafness. The paraparesis gradually or rapidly develops into a nearly complete paraplegia with bladder paralysis, and death is frequently caused by chronic urinary tract infection. The blood and CSF serological reactions are frequently (blood) or occasionally (CSF) positive but yaws and syphilis are common diseases in the population from which these cases arise. A histamine-fast achlorhydria is common in the cases. No therapeutic regime has yet shown convincing benefit except for the general non-specific measures of physiotherapy and rehabilitation.

Pathological findings.—The meninges around the brain and particularly those around the spinal cord are thickened and adherent. Histological sections show a low-grade leptomeningitis with a cellular exudate of lymphocytes with some plasma cells and macrophages. Within the spinal cord there is a similar perivascular lymphocytic inflammatory process affecting the grey matter by neuronal depletion and the white matter by a spongy degeneration. Long-tract degenerations in the corticospinal, gracile, and spino-cerebellar tracts is seen and this is presumably secondary to the direct cord damage. The spinal nerve roots and the optic and other cranial nerves are affected by a similar chronic inflammatory process. The pathological picture is very similar to that of the various forms of neurosyphilis but some features, e.g. endarteritis, are said to be absent. Spirochaetes have never been demonstrated in the necropsy material.

Etiology.—The etiology of this strange disease is so-far unknown. There are similarities to neurosyphilis, subacute combined degeneration of the spinal cord, lathyrism and nutritional myelopathy. Further investigation of these cases is required.

REFERENCES

TOXIC DISEASES

AHLBOM, H. E. (1941). The results of radiotherapy of hypopharyngeal cancer at the Radiumhemmet, Stockholm, 1930–1939. *Acta radiol. (Stockh.)*, **22**, 155–171.

ALEXANDER, L. (1938). Clinical and neuropathological aspects of electrical injuries. *J. indust. Hyg.*, **20**, 191–243.

ARING, C. D. (1942). The systemic nervous affinity of triorthocresyl phosphate (Jamaica ginger palsy). *Brain*, **65**, 34–47.

BECHAR, M., FREUD, M., KOTT, E., KOTT, I., KRAVVIC, H., STERN, J., SANDBANK, U. and BORNSTEIN, B. (1970). Hepatic cirrhosis with post-shunt myelopathy. *J. Neurol. Sci.*, **11**, 101–107.

BERRY, K. and OLSZEWSKI, J. (1963). Pathology of intrathecal phenol injection in man. *Neurology (Minneap.)*, **13**, 152–154.

BLANKENHORN, D. and WOLFF, H. G. (1948). Myelitis following the administration of neoarsphenamine. *J. lab. clin. Med.*, **33**, 1165–1168.

BODEN, G. (1948). Radiation myelitis of cervical spinal cord. *Brit. J. Radiol.*, **21**, 464–469.

BODEN, G. (1950). Radiation myelitis of brain-stem. *J. Fac. Radiol. (Lond.)*, **2**, 79–94.

BOEHME, D. H. (1971). Myelopathia saturnina. *Acta Neuropath. (Berl.)*, **18**, 356–360.

BUNGE, R. P. and SETTLAGE, H. (1957). Neurological lesions in cats following cerebrospinal fluid manipulation. *J. Neuropath. exp. Neurol.*, **16**, 471–491.

BURNS, R. J., JONES, A. N. and ROBERTSON, J. S. (1972). Pathology of radiation myelopathy. *J. Neurol. Neurosurg. Psychiat.*, **35**, 888–898.

CAVANAGH, J. B. (1954). Toxic effects of tri-ortho-cresyl phosphate on nervous system; experimental study in hens. *J. Neurol. Neurosurg. Psychiat.*, **17**, 163–172.

DASTUR, D. K. (1962). Lathyrism. Some aspects of the disease in man and animals. *World Neurol.*, **3**, 721–730.

DASTUR, D. K. and WADIA, N. H. (1969). Spinal meningitides with radiculo-myelopathy. Pt 2. Pathology and pathogenesis. *J. neurol. Sci.*, **8**, 261–297.

DYNES, J. B. and SMEDAL, M. I. (1960), Radiation myelitis. *Amer. J. Roentgenol.*, **83**, 78–87.

ELKINGTON, J. ST. C. (1936). Meningitis serosa circumscripta spinalis (spinal arachnoiditis). *Brain*, **59**, 181–203.

FLOREY, M. E. (1952). *The Clinical Application of Antibiotics*, pp. 20–21. London: Oxford Univ. Press.

FRENCH, J. D. (1947). Recurrent arachnoiditis in the dorsal spinal region. *Arch. Neurol. Psychiat. (Chic.)*, **58**, 200–206.

FRIEDE, R. L. and ROESSMANN, U. (1969). Destruction of peripheral white matter of the spinal cord, brain-stem, and optic tract. *J. Neurol. Neurosurg. Psychiat.*, **32**, 38–42.

GLASER, J. (1934). Clinical arsenical myelitis and neuritis due to acetarsone: report of two cases with one death; negative observations at necropsy. *Amer. J. Dis. Child.*, **48**, 134–148.

HAY, R. C., YONEZAWA, T. and DERRICK, W. S. (1959). Control of intractable pain in advanced cancer by subarachnoid alcohol block. *J. Amer. med. Ass.*, **169**, 1315–1320.

HENRY, P., CASTAIGNS, G., HOERNI, B. and TOUCHARD, J. (1971). La myélopathie progressive post-radiothérapeutique tardive. *J. neurol. Sci.*, **14**, 325–340.

HOWIESON, J. and MEGISON, L. C., Jr. (1968). Complications of vertebral artery catheterization. *Radiology*, **91**, 1109–1111.

HUGHES, J. T. and BROWNELL, B. (1965). Paraplegia following retrograde abdominal aortography. *Arch. Neurol. (Chic.)*, **12**, 650–657.

HURST, E. W. (1955). Adhesive arachnoiditis and vascular blockage caused by detergents and other chemical irritants: experimental study. *J. Path. Bact.*, **70**, 167–178.

ITABASHI, H. H., BEBIN, J. and DE JONG, R. N. (1957). Postirradiation cervical myelopathy: report of two cases. *Neurology* (*Minneap.*), **7**, 844–852.

JELLINGER, K. and STURM, K. W. (1971). Delayed radiation myelopathy in man. *J. neurol. Sci.*, **14**, 389–408.

KIDD, J. G. and LANGWORTHY, O. R. (1933). Jake paralysis; paralysis following ingestion of Jamaica ginger extract adulterated with tri-ortho-cresyl-phosphate. *Bull. Johns Hopk. Hosp.*, **52**, 39–64.

KILLEN, D. A. and FOSTER, J. H. (1960). Spinal cord injury as a complication of aortography. *Ann. Surg.*, **152**, 211–230.

KULOWSKI, J. and SCOTT, W. (1934). Localized adhesive spinal arachnoiditis. An obscure cause of radiating low back pain. *J. Bone Jt Surg.*, **16**, 699–703.

LANGWORTHY, O. R. (1932). Necrosis of the spinal cord produced by electrical injuries. *Bull. Johns Hopk. Hosp.*, **51**, 210–216.

LLOYD, J. W., HUGHES, J. T. and DAVIES-JONES, G. A. B. (1972). Relief of severe intractable pain by barbotage of cerebrospinal fluid. *Lancet*, **1**, 354–355.

LÖKEN, A. C. and HAYMAKER, W. (1949). Pamaquine poisoning in man, with clinicopathologic study of one case. *Amer. J. trop. Med.*, **29**, 341–352.

LYON, L. W. (1971). Transfemoral vertebral angiography as a cause of an anterior spinal artery syndrome. *J. Neurosurg.*, **35**, 328–330.

MAHALEY, M. S., Jr. and ODOM, G. L. (1966). Complication following intrathecal injection of fluorescein. *J. Neurosurg.*, **25**, 298–299.

MAHER, R. M. (1955). Relief of pain in incurable cancer. *Lancet*, **1**, 18–20.

MALAMUD, N., BOLDREY, E., WELCH, W. K. and FADELL, E. J. (1954). Necrosis of brain and spinal cord following X-ray therapy. *J. Neurosurg.*, **11**, 353–362.

MARGOLIS, G. (1970). Pathogenesis of contrast media injury: insight provided by neurotoxicity studies. *Invest. Radiol.*, **5**, 392–406.

MARGOLIS, G., TARAZI, A. K. and GRIMSON, K. S. (1956). Contrast medium injury to the spinal cord produced by aortography. *J. Neurosurg.*, **13**, 349–365.

NELSON, J. (1943). Intramedullary cavitation resulting from adhesive spinal arachnoiditis. *Arch. Neurol. Psychiat.* (*Chic.*), **50**, 1–7.

NIELSEN, J. M. (1952). Progressive course of arachnoiditis simulating syringomyelia. *Trans. Amer. neurol. Ass.*, **77**, 174–177.

PALLIS, C. A., LOUIS, S. and MORGAN, R. L. (1961). Radiation myelopathy. *Brain*, **84**, 460–479.

PALMER, J. J. (1972). Radiation myelopathy. *Brain*, **95**, 109–122.

PANT, S. S., REBEIZ, J. J. and RICHARDSON, E. P., Jr. (1968). Spastic paraparesis following portacaval shunts. *Neurology (Minneap.)*, **18**, 134–141.

PENTSCHEW, A. (1958). Intoxikationen. In *Handbuch der Speziellen Pathologischen Anatomie und Histologie*, Vol. XIII 2B, pp. 1907–2502. Ed. by W. Scholz. Berlin-Göttingen-Heidelberg: Springer.

PENTSCHEW, A. (1971). Introduction to Intoxications. Chap. 121 in *Pathology of the Nervous System*, Vol. 2. Ed. by J. Minckler. New York: McGraw-Hill.

PLUM, F. (1955). Myelitis and myelopathy. In *Clinical Neurology*, 2nd edit., pp. 1726–1727. Ed. by A. B. Baker. New York: Hoeber-Harper.

RÉTIF, J., BRIHAYE, J. and PÉRIER, O. (1964). L'arachnoïdite spinale. *Neuro-Chirurgie*, **10**, 370–386.

RICHTER, R. W. and ROSENBERG, R. N. (1968). Transverse myelitis associated with heroin addiction. *J. Amer. med. Ass.*, **206**, 1255–1257.

SANTOS, R. DOS, LAMAS, A. C. and CALDAS, J. (1929). A Arteriografia dos Membros. *Med. contemp.* **47**, 93–96.

SCHEIN, P. S., YESSAYAN, L. and MAYMAN, C. I. (1971). Acute transverse myelitis associated with intravenous opium. *Neurology (Minneap.)*, **21**, 101–102.

SCHULTZ, P. and SCHWARZ, G. A. (1970). Radiculomyelopathy following intrathecal instillation of methylene blue. *Arch. Neurol. (Chic.)*, **22**, 240–244.

SMITH, H. V. and SPALDING, J. M. K. (1959). Outbreak of paralysis in Morocco due to ortho-cresyl phosphate poisoning. *Lancet*, **2**, 1019–1021.

SMITH, M. I. and LILLIE, R. D. (1931). The histopathology of triortho-cresyl phosphate poisoning. *Arch. Neurol. Psychiat. (Chic.)*, **26**, 976–992.

STEVENSON, L. D. and ECKHARDT, R. E. (1945). Myelomalacia of the cervical portion of the spinal cord, probably the result of roentgen therapy. *Arch. Path.*, **39**, 109–112.

SWEET, K. K., DUMOFF-STANLEY, E., DOWLING, H. F. and LEPPER, M. H. (1945). The treatment of pneumococcic meningitis with penicillin. *J. Amer. med. Ass.*, **127**, 263–267.

TSUKAGOSHI, H., MORI, H., ENOMOTO, A., NAKAO, K. and FUKUSHIMA, N. (1970). Sensory polyradiculoneuropathy following spinal anesthesia. *Neurology (Minneap.)*, **20**, 266–274.

VONDERAHE, A. R. (1931). Pathologic changes in paralysis caused by drinking Jamaica ginger. *Arch. Neurol. Psychiat. (Chic.)*, **25**, 29–43.

WADIA, N. H. and DASTUR, D. K. (1969). Spinal meningitides with radiculo-myelopathy. Pt 1. Clinical and radiological features. *J. Neurol. Sci.*, **8**, 239–260.

WEISS, R. M., SWEENEY, L. and DREYFUSS, M. (1962). Circumscribed adhesive spinal arachnoiditis. *J. Neurosurg.*, **19**, 435–438.

WILCOCKS, C. and MANSON-BAHR, P. E. C. (1972). *Manson's Tropical Diseases*, 17th edit. London: Baillière Tindall.

WINKELMAN, N. W., GOTTEN, N. and SCHEIBERT, D. (1953). Localized adhesive spinal arachnoiditis. A study of twenty-five cases with reference to etiology. *Trans. Amer. neurol. Ass.*, **78**, 15–18.

DEFICIENCY DISEASES

BRAIN, W. R. (1947). Malnutrition of the nervous system. *Brit. med. J.*, **2**, 763–766.

DENNY-BROWN, D. (1947). Neurological conditions resulting from prolonged and severe dietary restriction. *Medicine (Baltimore)*, **26**, 41–113.

ERBSLÖH, F. (1958). Funikuläre Spinalerkrankung. In *Handbuch der Speziellen Pathologischen Anatomie und Histologie*, Vol. XIII/2B, pp. 1526–1601. Ed. by W. Scholz. Berlin-Göttingen-Heidelberg: Springer.

GRIEVE, S., JACOBSON, S. and PROCTOR, N. S. F. (1967). A nutritional myelopathy occurring in the Bantu on the Witwatersrand. *Neurology (Minneap.)*, **17**, 1205–1212.

MEYER, A. (1963). In *Greenfield's Neuropathology*, 2nd edit., pp. 288–323. Ed. by W. Blackwood, W. H. McMenemy, A, Meyer, R. M. Norman and D. S. Russell. London: Edward Arnold.

PANT, S. S., ASBURY, A. K. and RICHARDSON, E. P., Jr. (1968). The myelopathy of pernicious anemia. A neuropathological re-appraisal. *Acta. Neurol. Scand.*, **44**, Suppl. 35.

PENTSCHEW, A. (1958). Mangelzustände. In *Handbuch der Speziellen Pathologischen Anatomie und Histologie*, Vol. XIII/2B, pp. 2503–2570. Ed. by W. Scholz. Berlin-Göttingen-Heidelberg: Springer.

ROBERTSON, W. B. and CRUICKSHANK, E. K. (1972). Jamaican (tropical) myeloneuropathy. Chap. 178 in *Pathology of the Nervous System*, Vol. 3. Ed. by J. Minckler. New York: McGraw-Hill.

RUSSELL, J. S. R., BATTEN, F. E. and COLLIER, J. (1900). Subacute combined degeneration of the spinal cord. *Brain*, **23**, 39–110.

SPILLANE, J. D. (1947). *Nutritional Disorders of the Nervous System*. Edinburgh: Livingstone.

CHAPTER IX

DEMYELINATING DISEASES

At the present time it is impossible to classify, on an etiological basis, any of the diseases dealt with in this chapter, and even the term "demyelinating disease" is open to criticism. The name refers to the histological find of disproportionate loss of myelin compared with the axonal damage. This finding must not be interpreted too rigidly since in many of these cases axon damage may be in certain areas quite extensive. Also in some diseases of quite different behaviour, e.g. subacute combined degeneration, demyelination is evident. Other features should be taken into consideration. These diseases primarily affect white matter, the lesions are widely disseminated throughout the brain and spinal cord, and in the early stages are seen to be situated perivenously. Poser (1968) has reviewed this whole group of diseases.

Multiple Sclerosis

This disease is the example *par excellence* of a demyelinating disease. The first illustrations of the pathological lesions of multiple sclerosis are to be found in the atlases of Cruveilhier (1835–42) and Carswell (1838). Among the early pathological reports are many German contributions notably those of Rokitansky, Leyden, Rindfleish and Zenker. Charcot (1868) deservedly is credited with the recognition of the salient clinical features and the important pathological findings. The world literature on the subject is now of enormous dimensions and here one can only select a few important pathological reports, Bielschowsky (1903), Dawson (1916), Jakob (1929), Schaltenbrand (1943) and Zimmerman and Netsky (1950). The reader is recommended to the reviews of Peters (1958*a*), Greenfield and Norman (1963), Lumsden (1955, 1964), and Peters (1968).

Age, sex, and geographical incidence.—In most published series the commonest age of onset is given as the second or third decade. The sex incidence has varied and there is no constant finding. The geographical incidence has attracted considerable attention. The diseases appears commoner in temperate climates and the incidence increases as one moves further from the equator.

Clinical course.—A detailed account would be out of place here. The cardinal feature is episodic neurological symptoms and signs indicative of multiple foci of white matter damage. The relapses and remissions of the disease are unique in neurological diseases. The spinal cord is one of the commonest regions affected; some cases, presenting difficulty in diagnosis clinically, have only spinal-cord involvement and in others this feature predominates.

Pathological findings outside the spinal cord.—No abnormal findings have been consistently observed outside the nervous system. The plaques in the cerebrum and brain stem are similar in nature to those in the spinal cord. In a survey of their distribution in the cerebrum, Brownell and Hughes (1963) found them in every anatomical structure. The favoured sites were the walls of the lateral ventricles and the junction of the cortex and white matter.

Pathological findings in the spinal cord.—Macroscopically the spinal cord is usually atrophied and this is very likely in a chronic case and one in which the spinal cord is predominantly affected. The leptomeninges may be thickened and opaque. Where the plaques involve the surface of the cord, they are faintly seen as circumscribed dark areas. They are easily seen on transverse slicing after fixation. Plaques appear to occur at any segmental level of the cord.

Microscopically, the size, shape, and position of the plaques are more easily seen. They are best examined in a myelin stain (Fig. 56) such as Weil's stain together with a glial stain, such as Holzer, to demonstrate the gliosis. Fog (1950) studied the topography of the lesions which, in his series, occurred commonly in certain areas. These were the centre of each posterior column, in the centre and posterior two-thirds of the lateral columns, and in the anterior columns symmetrically on both sides of the anterior median fissure. Fog considered the plaques were primarily related to the spinal veins and their drainage territories.

The detailed histology of a plaque is similar both in the brain and in the spinal cord. In sections stained for myelin there is a sharply defined irregular myelin loss, usually complete and replaced by fibrous gliosis. The oligodendroglia disappear with the myelin, nuclei are few, and only moderate numbers of plump well-spaced fibrous astrocytes are seen. The edge of the plaque may be active with microglial proliferation and breaking-down

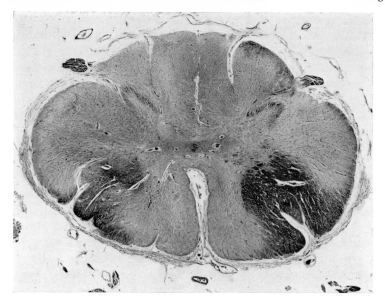

FIG. 56.—Transverse section, stained for myelin, at C2 segmented level of, a spinal cord severely involved by multiple sclerosis. Plaques have involved almost the whole cross-sectional area at this level. Weil ×9.

myelin. Axons can usually be seen in the plaques but these may be distorted. Neurone cell bodies seem completely unchanged when the plaque involves grey matter. Wallerian degeneration above and below the lesions is usually slight; certainly it is very much less than in any other severe spinal cord disorder. This would agree with a disease which tends to spare the axons.

The above description is of typical cases and describes the middle period of the disease. Some cases have multiple early cellular lesions and these cases are difficult to separate nosologically from acute disseminated encephalomyelitis. The very chronic cases are also atypical. The whole spinal cord is, in these cases, atrophied and in the transverse sections there is so much confluent demyelination and Wallerian degeneration that distinct plaques cannot readily be demonstrated.

Acute Disseminated Encephalomyelitis (Acute Perivascular Myelinoclasis)

This interesting disease (which it is current practice to include in the demyelinating diseases) occurs following a variety of acute infectious diseases such as smallpox, vaccinia, varicella, measles and influenza. It may occur spontaneously and a similar condition has been provoked by courses of anti-rabic treatment. The considerable interest of this disease has been enhanced by the success of experimental workers in producing acute encephalomyelitis by the injection of homologous nervous tissue. The earliest reports of this success in monkeys by Rivers and Schwentker (1935) and Ferraro and Jarvis (1940), came under suspicion of referring to lesions of spontaneous demyelinating conditions. Later work has amply shown these suspicions to be unjustified. The difficulties in producing the experimental condition were enormously reduced following the work on adjuvants by Freund and McDermott (1942). Using similar adjuvants Kabat et al. (1947) reported the rapid production of acute encephalitis in monkeys by injection of brain tissue with adjuvants. In a subsequent paper, Kabat et al. (1949) reported a convincing autoimmune experiment by successfully using a monkey's own brain tissue removed by frontal lobectomy. Acute disseminated encephalomyelitis and experimental allergic encephalomyelitis have been extensively studied in the hope that the knowledge gained would have a wider application to the problem of multiple sclerosis. But as we shall see there are important differences both in the clinical and pathological features of these conditions.

Clinical course.—Despite the variety of preceding illnesses the subsequent encephalomyelitis, occurring usually after an interval of approximately 10 days, has a remarkably constant course. The so-called "primary" cases may similarly follow an unidentified virus infection. Very rarely there is a myelitis without signs of encephalitis. Henneaux and Delcourt (1954) described such a case following vaccination and Amyot (1957) described a case following mumps. These cases did not have necropsy studies but the author has verified at necropsy a case that followed vaccination, in which myelitis was the only lesion.

Pathological findings.—The changes in brain and spinal cord are alike and were described in detail by Turnbull and McIntosh (1926) in their post-vaccinial cases. The essential feature is the sleeving of the cerebral venules with a zone of congestion and partial softening. Other changes are lymphocytic and plasma-cell infiltration of the Virchow-Robin spaces and proliferation of the reticulum cells in the adventitia of the veins. These latter changes are less constant than the perivenular sleeving from which Marsden and Hurst (1932) proposed the name "acute perivascular myelino-clasis". The appearance in myelin-stained sections is a spotty state of the white matter (Fig. 57). In some areas the lesions coalesce into large regions of necrosis. As we have observed, the basic pathology is that of white matter necrosis and there is no true demyelination.

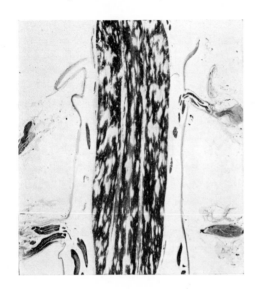

FIG. 57.—Longitudinal section, stained for myelin, of the spinal cord from a case of acute disseminated encephalomyelitis. Weil × 3.

Studies of the immune mechanism at work in acute disseminated encephalomyelitis and in the comparable experimental allergic encephalomyelitis have shown that the lymphocytic cellular exudate is the key to the understanding of the disease. The lymphocytes, which figure so prominently in the cellular reaction, are part of a cell-mediated hypersensitivity reaction directed against myelin.

Neuromyelitis Optica (Devic's Disease)

In 1870 Clifford Allbutt, then a physician at Leeds Infirmary, published his observations on the ophthalmoscopy of patients with acute myelitis. In one case optic neuritis supervened 12 weeks after the spinal lesion, and this report appears to be the first which records this association. Allbutt's case did not come to autopsy and the first pathological observations were made by Dreschfield (1882) a physician at the Manchester Royal Infirmary and Professor of Pathology. He reported two autopsied cases of acute myelitis with optic neuritis. He noted softening in the spinal cord and demyelination in the optic nerves. The eponymous use of Devic's name refers to the latter's report in 1894. Addressing the French Congress of Medicine at Lyons, he presented a case and reviewed 16 previous reports. His pupil Gault expanded these observations in a doctorate thesis. Devic's case is particularly interesting because in addition to the severe lesion of the spinal cord and optic nerves, cerebral foci of demyelination were present. When Goulden (1914) reviewed the literature he found 51 case reports to which he added a case with autopsy studies. In discussing the autopsy reports of 14 cases he noted the frequency with which demyelination proceeded to necrosis with destruction of nerve fibres. He thought that infiltration with round cells was common but neuroglial proliferation was scanty. The next full review of the literature was made by Beck (1927) who added his own case report to a review of 70 cases. His case showed massive demyelination of the spinal cord and optic nerves. Four types of cellular reaction were present: perivascular round-cell infiltration, capillary proliferation, neuroglial proliferation and polymorpho-nuclear-cell infiltration. Stansbury (1949) added five autopsied case reports to an extensive review of approximately 200 cases. In a doctorate thesis (Hughes, 1961) I have presented the necropsy findings of several relevant cases and reviewed the subject. For a detailed review the reader is referred to Peters (1958b).

We may summarise the reported pathological findings as follows:

The lesions of neuromyelitis optica are found in the optic pathway, spinal cord, and brain stem, occasionally in the cerebrum, but very rarely in the cerebellum. They are characterised histologically by demyelination but often with destruction of axis cylinders. There is a distinct tendency to necrosis and cavity formation particularly seen in the spinal cord. Marked proliferation of microglia occurs but there is only a moderate astrocytic reaction. Perivascular cellular infiltration is often present, usually lymphocytic, but plasma cells and rarely polymorphonuclear leucocytes may be present.

Whilst it is possible to regard the association of acute myelitis with optic neuritis as a clinical syndrome, the author is unconvinced of its reality as a distinct pathological entity. We have mentioned the cerebral foci in Devic's original case. Similar but more extensive cerebral involvement occurred in Case 3 of the report by Stewart *et al.* (1927), whose case had features of diffuse sclerosis and neuromyelitis optica. Confusion of neuromyelitis optica with multiple sclerosis has certainly occurred. Van Bogaert (1927) presented a case of neuromyelitis optica to the Paris Neurological Society and in 1932 he reported the autopsy of the same case which now he interpreted as multiple sclerosis (Van Bogaert, 1932). That some of the older reported cases have been due to syphilis is probable. The case of Laruelle and Goudissart (1930) had a positive Wassermann reaction, and they found, in reviewing 20 case reports, serological evidence of syphilis in five. To these causes of possible diagnostic confusion the author would add subacute combined degeneration, since in this disease there may be an associated optic neuritis.

It is doubtful whether a single pathological basis exists for the disease entity neuromyelitis optica. However the coincidence of a lesion in the optic nerve with a lesion in the spinal cord still requires explanation even though a variety of primary causes may be evident. Possibly the common factor is the rigidity of the optic nerve canal and of the spinal canal. Swelling, from optic neuritis and a coincident demyelinating plaque in the spinal cord, may cause much more damage in these locations with a consequent emphasis on the two components of the syndrome neuromyelitis optica.

What is beyond doubt is that many of the cases so diagnosed on clinical grounds will prove at autopsy to have some other condition such as multiple sclerosis. There remain a few pathological reports not easily reconciled with any other diagnosis. In this the pathology in the spinal cord is the same as the next condition to be described.

Acute Necrotic Myelopathy

This is a rare condition of primary necrosis of the spinal cord which at necropsy has very distinctive features. These cases have been reported under a variety of names: myelomalacia by Bassoe and Hassin (1921), acute necrotic myelitis by Greenfield and Turner (1939), acute necrotic myelopathy by Hoffman (1955) and myelitis necroticans diffusa by Kahle and Schaltenbrand (1955). Reviews of this condition were made by Moersch and Kernohan (1934), Jaffe and Freeman (1943) and Hughes (1961). In this last mentioned work I reviewed from the literature

20 well-documented cases with necropsies and added five autopsied cases showing the acute, subacute and chronic pathological findings.

Clinical course.—There is no particular sex or age incidence and no cases have shown any familial tendency. Some cases have had optic neuritis and one (Hughes, 1961) had coexistent multiple sclerosis. Sometimes the disease is ushered in with an upper respiratory infection.

The first neurological symptoms are usually those of sensory disturbance, following which weakness develops. The paresis, initially of upper motor neurone type, rapidly becomes a flaccid, areflexic paralysis. At the same time sensory loss, corresponding to the affected spinal cord segments, becomes complete. The course of the neurological disease is always short, being numbered in days. After this period, no neurological improvement occurs, nor is there any further extension of the spinal cord disease. The cerebrospinal fluid shows an increase of cells, which initially are polymorphs, a rise in protein, and the presence of globulin.

Pathological findings.—These vary according to the length of time that the disease is survived. Hughes (1961) recognised early, intermediate and late stages. In the first two weeks, the cord is swollen and softer than normal (Fig. 58a, b). The cut surface on transverse section appears opaque and already the extent of the affected tissue is apparent. The white matter is predominantly affected and the preservation of the grey matter is striking. The spinal cord vessels and meninges appear entirely normal.

Microscopically, the first change is swelling of individual myelin tubes. What appears to be a further stage is the development in the white matter of a striking spongy appearance, which at high-power magnification is seen to be formed by disintegration of myelin tubes. The spaces are usually empty but sometimes with silver stains swollen axonic material can be seen either as droplets or as terminal club-like expansions of damaged nerve fibres. In this early stage there are perivascular lymphocytes and monocytes and an abundance of proliferating microglia. These changes affect primarily the white matter and the grey columns are strikingly preserved.

The course of this disease often proceeds to death from intercurrent infection within three to twelve months and this "intermediate" stage is that to which the descriptions of most reported cases apply (Fig. 59a, b). The affected region of the spinal cord

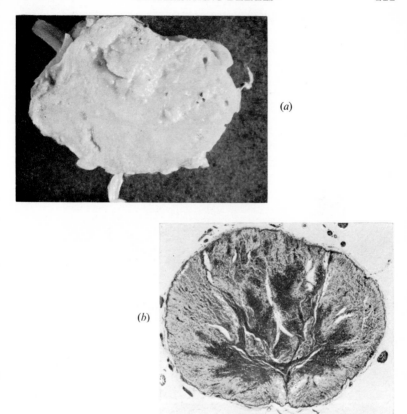

(a)

(b)

FIG. 58a.—Acute phase of acute necrotic myelopathy. Survival 4 weeks. Photograph ×4 of T12 spinal cord segment where the whole cross-section of the spinal cord shows softening. The microscopical appearance at this level is seen in Fig. 58b.

FIG. 58b.—Transverse section at T12 stained for myelin. Extensive white matter destruction has occurred but the architecture of the grey matter is still preserved. Weil ×4.

is swollen and is now extremely soft to palpation. Without the containing pia-arachnoid the cord would collapse, and transverse cuts through the worst affected region show semi-liquid cord substance. The form of the softened region is that of a long spindle, mainly a fusiform region of softening affecting the whole of many consecutive spinal cord segments and ending above and below by tapering in the course of one or two segments to a small area in the posterior columns. This unusual shape has been

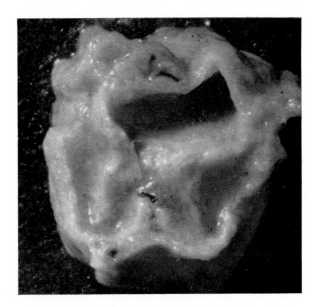

FIG. 59a.—Intermediate phase of acute necrotic myelopathy. Survival 6 months. Photograph ×9 of T9 spinal cord segment cut transversely. There is gross softening with liquefaction of the white matter. The microscopical appearance at this level is seen in Fig. 59b.

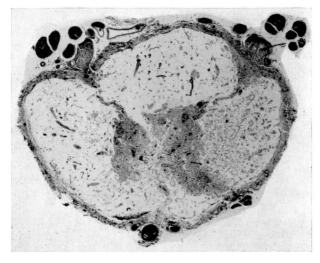

FIG. 59b.—Transverse section at T9 stained for myelin. The white matter destruction is complete but the architecture of the grey matter is preserved. Note the myelin remaining in the posterior nerve roots. Weil ×9.

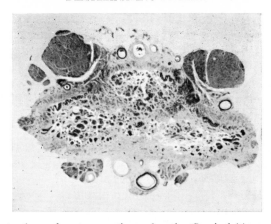

FIG. 60.—Late phase of acute necrotic myelopathy. Survival 14 years. Transverse section at L1 stained for myelin. No normal spinal cord remains, instead there are bundles of interlacing myelinated nerve fibres cut in transverse section. Note the plump posterior nerve roots from which the abnormal bundles of nerve fibres arise. The anterior nerve roots are atrophied since their parent cell bodies have perished. Weil × 12.

reported in several of the cases in the literature but also is seen in traumatic myelopathy. A recurrent feature noted during exploratory operations on these cases has been swelling of the spinal cord and such swelling, being restricted by the meninges, may force softened spinal-cord tissue upwards and downwards at the point of least mechanical resistance. This region may be in the centre of the posterior columns thus accounting for the ends of the spindle.

The microscopical appearance in this intermediate stage is simple, since only loose lipid phagocytes can be made out among necrotic debris. A peripheral rim of lipid phagocytes is supported by the pia-arachnoid. The necrosis is extreme and all other cellular structures including vessels, astrocytes and oligodendroglia have perished.

In the late stages after ten or twelve years (Hughes, 1961) the spinal cord shows an extreme degree of atrophy over a large number of consecutive cord segments. The meninges and vessels are normal. Microscopically, in the atrophied spinal cord segments, normal white and grey matter is absent. The space is replaced by bundles of nerve fibres intertwined longitudinally in groups of ten to twenty fibres (Fig. 60). The nerve fibres are myelinated and have adjacent nuclei like those of the cells of

Schwann. The source of these fibres is apparent when we examine the spinal nerve roots. The anterior roots are completely atrophied since their cell bodies in the anterior horns are destroyed. By contrast, the posterior roots are relatively plump and contain many nerve fibres which enter the cord and join the interwoven abnormal nerve bundles. The significance of this phenomenon was discussed by Hughes and Brownell (1963).

Etiology of acute necrotic myelopathy.—This is at the moment quite unknown but from a study of the available necropsy observations, I am inclined to place these cases among the demyelinating diseases. Of the five cases that I have studied intensively, one had previous optic neuritis whilst one had plaques of multiple sclerosis in the cerebrum, brain stem and optic tract. The other suggested causes are vascular obstruction, infective agents and toxic agents. The distribution of the spinal cord lesion is unlike any arterial distribution or venous drainage. No major cause of arterial obstruction has ever been demonstrated and cases of spinal thrombophlebitis have a subacute necrotic myelitis of a different kind. No infective or toxic agent has ever been convincingly proven, though in such a rare disease, it is difficult to amass sufficient observations to exclude the possibility of the action of such agents.

REFERENCES

MULTIPLE SCLEROSIS

BIELSCHOWSKY, M. (1903). Zur Histologie der multiplen sklerose; Untersuchgsergebnisse neuer Methoden. *Neurol. Zbl.*, **22**, 770–777.

BROWNELL, B. and HUGHES, J. T. (1963). The distribution of plaques in the cerebrum in multiple sclerosis. *J. Neurol. Neurosurg. Psychiat.*, **25**, 315–320.

CARSWELL, R. (1838). *Pathological Anatomy, Illustrations of the Elementary Forms of Disease*, Plate IV. London: Longman.

CHARCOT, J. M. (1868). Leçons sur Les Maladies Chroniques du Système nerveux. *Gaz. Hôp.* (*Paris*), **41**, 405–406, 409.

CRUVEILHIER, J. (1835–42). *Anatomie pathologique du corps humain*, Vol. 2. Paris: Baillière.

DAWSON, J. W. (1916). The histology of disseminated sclerosis. *Edinb. med. J.*, **16**, 229–241.

FOG, T. (1950). Topographic distribution of plaques in spinal cord in multiple sclerosis. *Arch. Neurol. Psychiat.* (*Chic.*), **63**, 382–414.

GREENFIELD, J. G. and NORMAN, R. M. (1963). In *Greenfield's Neuro-*

pathology, 2nd edit., pp. 475–519. Ed. by W. Blackwood, W. H. McMenemy, A. Meyer, R. M. Norman and D. S. Russell. London: Edward Arnold.

JAKOB, A. (1929). *Specielle Histopathologie des Grosshirns.* Wien: Deuticke.

LUMSDEN, C. E. (1955). In *Multiple Sclerosis*, by McAlpine, D., Compston, N. D., and Lumsden, C. E. Edinburgh: Livingstone.

LUMSDEN, C. E. (1964). In *Multiple Sclerosis, A Reappraisal*, by McAlpine, D., Lumsden, C. E. and Acheson, E. D. Edinburgh: Livingstone.

PETERS, G. (1958a). Multiple Sklerose. In *Handbuch der Speziellen Pathologischen Anatomie und Histologie.* Vol. XIII/2A, pp. 525–602. Ed. by W. Scholz. Berlin-Göttingen-Heidelberg: Springer.

PETERS, G. (1968). Multiple Sclerosis. In *Pathology of the Nervous System*, Vol. 1. Ed. by J. Minckler. New York: McGraw-Hill.

POSER, C. M. (1968). Diseases of the myelin sheath. In *Pathology of the Nervous System*, Vol. 1. Ed. by J. Minckler. New York: McGraw-Hill.

SCHALTENBRAND, G. (1943). *Die multiple Sklerose des Menschen.* Leipzig: Thieme.

ZIMMERMAN, H. M. and NETSKY, M. G. (1950). The pathology of multiple sclerosis. *Res. Publ. Ass. nerv. ment. Dis.*, **28**, 271–312.

ACUTE DISSEMINATED ENCEPHALOMYELITIS

AMYOT, R. (1957). La myélite transverse d'étiologie ourlienne. Transverse myelitis following mumps. *Un. méd. Can.*, **86**, 941–948.

FERRARO, A. and JARVIS, G. A. (1940). Experimental disseminated encephalopathy in the monkey. *Arch. Neurol. Psychiat. (Chic.)*, **43**, 195–209.

FREUND, J. and McDERMOTT, J. (1942). Sensitisation to horse serum by means of adjuvants. *Proc. Soc. exp. Biol. (N.Y.)*, **49**, 548–553.

HENNEAUX, J. and DELCOURT, J. (1954). Myélite transverse consecutive à une vaccination anti-variolique. *Acta. neurol. belg.*, **54**, 449–456.

KABAT, E. A., WOLF, A. and BEZER, A. E. (1947). The rapid production of acute disseminated encephalomyelitis in rhesus monkeys by injection of heterologous and homologous brain tissue with adjuvants. *J. exp. Med.*, **85**, 117–129.

KABAT, E. A., WOLF, A. and BEZER, A. E. (1949). Studies on acute disseminated encephalomyelitis produced experimentally in rhesus monkeys; disseminated encephalomyelitis produced in monkeys with their own brain tissue. *J. exp. Med.*, **89**, 395–398.

MARSDEN, J. P. and HURST, E. W. (1932). Acute perivascular myelinoclasis (acute disseminated encephalomyelitis) in smallpox. *Brain*, **55**, 181–225.

RIVERS, T. M. and SCHWENTKER, F. F. (1935). Encephalomyelitis accompanied by myelin destruction experimentally produced in monkeys. *J. exp. Med.*, **61**, 689–702.

TURNBULL, H. M. and MCINTOSH, J. (1926). Encephalomyelitis following vaccination. *Brit. J. exp. Path.*, **7**, 181–222.

NEUROMYELITIS OPTICA

BECK, N. (1927). A case of diffuse myelitis associated with optic neuritis. *Brain*, **50**, 687–703.

BOGAERT, L. VAN (1927). Neuro-myélite optique aiguë avec dissociation albuminocytologic du liquide céphalo-rachidien. *J. Neurol. (Brux.)* **27**, 106–107.

BOGAERT, L. VAN (1932). Erreur de diagnostic: neuromyélite optique aiguë, premier stade d'une sclérose en plaque typique. *J. Neurol. (Brux.)*, **32**, 234–247.

DRESCHFIELD, J. (1882). On two cases of acute myelitis associated with optic neuritis. *Lancet*, **1**, 8, 52–53.

GOULDEN, C. (1914). Optic neuritis and myelitis. *Trans. ophthal. Soc. U.K.*, **34**, 229–252.

HUGHES, J. T. (1961). *Acute Idiopathic Myelomalacia*. (M.D. thesis). Victoria Univ. of Manchester.

LARUELLE, L. and GOUDISSART, P. (1930). Un cas de neuromyélite optique. *J. Neurol. (Brux.)*, **30**, 91–97.

PETERS, G. (1958b). Neuromyelitis optica. In *Handbuch der Speziellen Pathologischen Anatomie und Histologie*, Vol. XIII/2A, pp. 630–644. Ed. by W. Scholz. Berlin-Göttingen-Heidelberg: Springer.

STANSBURY, F. C. (1949). Neuromyelitis optica (Devic's disease); presentation of 5 cases, with pathologic study, and review of literature. *Arch. Ophthal.*, **42**, 292–335, 465–501.

STEWART, T. G., GREENFIELD, J. G. and BLANDY, M. A. (1927). Encephalitis periaxialis diffusa. Report of three cases with pathological examinations. *Brain*, **50**, 1–29.

ACUTE NECROTIC MYELOPATHY

BASSOE, P. and HASSIN, G. B. (1921). Myelitis and myelomalacia: a clinico-pathological study with remarks on the fate of gitter cells. *Arch. Neurol. Psychiat. (Chic.)*, **6**, 32–43.

GREENFIELD, J. G. and TURNER, J. W. A. (1939). Acute and subacute necrotic myelitis. *Brain*, **62**, 227–252.

HOFFMANN, H. L. (1955). Acute necrotic myelopathy. *Brain*, **78**, 377–393.

HUGHES, J. T. (1961). *Acute Idiopathic Myelomalacia*. (M.D. thesis). Victoria Univ. of Manchester.

HUGHES, J. T. and BROWNELL, B. (1963). Aberrant nerve fibres within the spinal cord. *J. Neurol. Neurosurg. Psychiat.*, **26**, 528–534.

JAFFE, D. and FREEMAN, W. (1943). Spinal necrosis and softening of obscure origin. *Arch. Neurol. Psychiat. (Chic.)*, **49**, 683–707.

KAHLE, W. and SCHALTENBRAND, G. (1955). Zur Klinik und Pathologie der Myelitis necroticans diffusa. *Dtsch. Z. Nervenheilk.*, **173**, 234–266.

MOERSCH, F. P. and KERNOHAN, J. W. (1934). Progressive necrosis of the spinal cord. *Arch. Neurol. Psychiat. (Chic.)*, **31**, 504–526.

CHAPTER X

TUMOURS

This historical development of our knowledge of tumours affecting the spinal cord can be traced back to the eighteenth century. Morgagni (1761) described paralysis caused by compression by tumour and Phillips (1792) described a primary tumour of the spinal cord. In the remarkable pathological atlas of Cruveilhier (1835–42) there is an illustration of a spinal-cord tumour and several case reports were mentioned by Ollivier (1837). There are many other notable reports but for mankind the most important event took place in 1887. In this year Sir William Gowers diagnosed an intradural tumour which was successfully removed by Sir Victor Horsley (Gowers and Horsley, 1888).

Recent additions to our knowledge of tumour etiology are eroding the boundaries between neoplastic and non-neoplastic diseases. In particular the virus has established its place alongside agents such as chemical carcinogens and X-rays as a proven cause of malignant neoplastic processes. At some future date it may be both possible and convenient to classify tumours etiologically, but in the foreseeable future their separation according to cell type will remain the most useful. Bailey and Cushing (1926) suggested such a classification of central nervous tissue tumours which, with only slight modifications, is in general use today. For current accounts the reader is referred to Kernohan and Sayre (1952), Henschen (1955), and Russell and Rubinstein (1971),

In considering tumours which affect the spinal cord we must first make an anatomical separation into intramedullary tumours and extramedullary tumours. The latter may arise from the meninges or nerve roots, or may be primary or secondary neoplasms involving the bony spinal canal. In all these different situations neoplasms have distinctive clinical and pathological features. Tumours of the conus medullaris and filum terminale are grouped with intramedullary tumours, but may differ in several respects from their cephalic counterparts.

It is easy to understand the damage caused to the spinal cord in the intramedullary tumours since in this group there is direct destruction by tumour. The damage may range from the slowly progressive infiltration of a diffuse astrocytoma to the rapid destruction caused by a secondary carcinoma. In the extramedullary tumours, the mechanism of the damage to the spinal cord varies and may be complex. The commonest effect is pressure and this may be exerted simply by a tumour such as a meningioma or neurofibroma growing in the spinal canal, or tumour infiltration of the spine may cause vertebral collapse with angulation. The effect of pressure in these cases is a subject which was discussed by Elsberg (1941) who had immense experience of the neurosurgical problem of cord compression. At any early stage there is interference with venous return and at operation there are small and empty veins at the region of compression changing to enlarged tortuous veins distended with blood below the tumour. At a later stage the circulation of spinal fluid in the subarachnoid space is blocked and the pulsation of the cord with heart respiration is abolished in the compressed region. Finally there is irreversible damage to the cord, a late stage in slowly growing tumours when nerve fibres have been severely compressed and the arterial blood supply is impeded.

This short account, summarised from the writings of Elsberg, and in agreement with several neurosurgical texts, assigns the greatest rôle in cord compression to a disturbance of the blood supply. The experimental work of Tarlov (1957) has questioned this view, at least for acute cord compression, which he could mimic in his experiments. It will be convenient to consider this experimental work here although in its clinical application it is more relevant to acute cord compression such as may develop following trauma.

Experimental Spinal Cord Compression

Tarlov (1957, 1972) has in dogs produced graded amounts of spinal cord compression induced both rapidly, analogous with a traumatic lesion, and more slowly, in an attempt to reproduce the gradually developing compression of a spinal tumour.

Rapid spinal cord compression.—Tarlov produced acute spinal cord compression by the rapid inflation of rubber balloons introduced into the extradural space of his dogs. In these experiments with rapid compression the effect produced depended on the amount of the compressing force and the duration of its action. By inflating the balloon to its fullest extent the maximal compressing force was applied and the effect on the unanaesthetised dog was the immediate loss simultaneously of all motor power and all forms of sensation. If this maximal compressing force was maintained for only one minute, then full neurological recovery was possible. Recovery was inconstant or incomplete if the pressure was maintained for more than one minute and, if five minutes pressure was exceeded, the full neurological recovery never occurred. If the compressive force was reduced to that just sufficient to produce sensorimotor paralysis, then recovery was possible after up to two hours compression.

Gradual spinal cord compression.—Tarlov produced gradual spinal cord compression by devices which slowly inflated the balloons over a period of days. He found that, as in the rapid compression experiments, the amount of compressing force applied affected the recovery of neurological function. When gradually increasing compression was applied to the point of total paralysis and then held at this compressive force, then about a week of compression could be survived with recovery of neurological function.

Mechanism of compression-produced paralysis.—It is of the greatest importance, in the management of human cases, to ascribe correctly the cause of spinal-compression paralysis either to mechanical destruction of spinal cord tissue or to an ischaemic effect produced by the pressure. Tarlov's work suggested that in his experiments mechanical pressure was the vital factor. The evidence for this was that the time of onset and rapidity of recovery from spinal compression differs from the time of onset and the rapidity of recovery from lesions known to be ischaemic. Compression paralysis occurs immediately the compressing force is applied, whilst ischaemic paralysis takes from one to five minutes to develop. The recovery from compressive paralysis may be delayed in its onset for several days whilst recovery from spinal cord ischaemia begins in a few minutes and is usually complete in an hour. The histological appearances of spinal cord compression and those of spinal cord ischaemia are different in that the ischaemic mechanisms affect predominantly the spinal grey column, whilst the compression lesions affect varying places of the spinal cord. Tarlov believes that in spinal-cord compression the most important factor is mechanical pressure on nervous tissue. He considers this is the explanation of sensorimotor paralysis in both acute and chronic spinal cord compression.

INTRAMEDULLARY TUMOURS

The most recent account is that of Slooff *et al.* (1964) who have analysed an unrivalled series of personally studied case reports collected at the Mayo Clinic over a period of 45 years. As in other series, ependymomas and astrocytomas make up the bulk of cases with all other tumours rare. Their 301 cases classified according to histological types were as follows:

Astrocytoma	86
Ependymoma	169
Oligodendroglioma	8
Mixed Glioma	3
Subependymal Glioma	1
Polar Spongioblastoma	1
Vascular Tumours	10
Sarcoma	1
Epidermoid and Dermoid Cysts	8
Teratoma	2
Lipoma	6
Neurilemmoma	1
Unclassified	1
Von Recklinghausen's disease with intramedullary tumours	4
	301

Astrocytoma

Slooff *et al.* (1964) found that astrocytomas of the spinal cord formed 3.05 per cent of all astrocytomas of the central nervous system. This was in close agreement with the expected figure calculated from the weight of the spinal cord which forms 2.57 per cent of the total weight of the central nervous system. They occur in all parts of the spinal cord, which may be involved throughout a considerable longitudinal extent. In most series there is a slight predominance of male cases.

Macroscopical appearance.—There is usually a fusiform expansion of the spinal cord (Fig. 61) which may obliterate the subdural and subarachnoid spaces. The cut surface is usually firm and grey but the rarer malignant examples may show yellow necrosis and

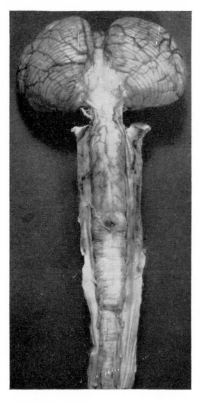

FIG. 61.—Glioblastoma producing cylindrical expansion of the cervical region of the spinal cord.

haemorrhage. Cystic degeneration is common; the most usual content being a yellow protein-rich fluid. Syringomyelia-like cavities may also be present.

Microscopical appearance.— In a large series such as that of Slooff *et al.* (1964) all the microscopical grades 1–4 of astrocytoma, distinguished by Mabon *et al* (1969), may be encountered. Grades 3 and 4 correspond to glioblastoma multiforme, used in the classification preferred by Russell and Rubinstein (1971). The microscopical features vary in each grade. The more slowly growing grade 1 tumours predominate; these usually are of fibrillary type with numerous astrocyte fibrils radiating in all directions from the spaced cell bodies and intertwining to form an indistinct mossy background. A common feature of these tumours are Rosenthal fibres, carrot-shaped thick fibres homogeneously staining with eosin or PTAH. In tumours of grades 2 and 3 the fibrillary tumours are more cellular and protoplasmic and gemistocytic types occur. The vessels may show endothelial proliferation. The grade 4 astrocytomas are rare; they may invade meninges and show haemorrhage and necrosis as in the cerebrum. The rapidly growing edge of these tumours may be relatively well demarcated from normal spinal cord (Fig. 62). Mitotic figures are present in moderate numbers (one per high power field) in grade 3 tumours and are abundant in those of grade 4 (Fig. 63).

Ependymoma

Ependymomas occur in the spinal cord and filum terminale rather more frequently than astrocytomas and considering the

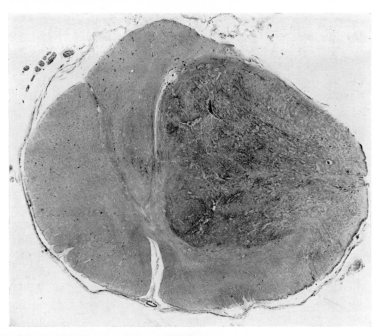

FIG. 62.—Transverse section of spinal cord segment C2 showing a malignant tumour (glioblastoma) on the left. The remaining cord is here infiltrated with astrocytoma. Holmes ×6.

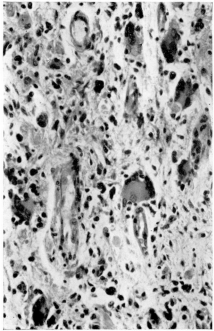

FIG. 63.—Photomicrograph at greater enlargement of the case seen in Fig. 62. Multinucleated giant cells are commonly seen in glioblastoma. Haematoxylin and eosin ×200.

small amount of ependymal tissue at risk, this must have a significant tendency for neoplasia. A very large number of these tumours occur in the caudal part of the cord and particularly in the filum terminale. As in astrocytoma, there is a slight male preponderance.

Macroscopical appearance.—The tumours within the spinal cord cause a fusiform expansion, usually more localised than in astro-cytomas. The tumours of the filum terminale are in the shape of an ovoid nodule expanding or attached to the filum. The tumours are soft and on cut surface have a homogeneous grey appearance often with small cysts. The intramedullary examples are often well demarcated from the surrounding spinal cord, even with a pseudo capsule; those of the filum are usually free among the cauda equina. These features are those of benign tumours; occasional examples are infiltrative, growing into meninges and even bone, whilst the cauda equina nerve roots may in these instances be matted together by tumour.

Microscopical appearance.—As with the astrocytomas, Mabon *et al.* (1949) have defined four grades of malignancy in ependy-momas. In addition to these malignancy grades, which correspond to degree of dedifferentiation, these authors recognise cellular, papillary and epithelial types of tumour. In the common cellular type of tumour there is a mosaic appearance with ependymal tumour cells set in an eosinophilic background of their fibrillar processes. The nuclei are conspicuous, being round or oval and of large size bounded by a distinct membrane (Fig. 64). In contrast, the cytoplasmic boundaries may be indistinct, forming a mossy background enhancing the mosaic patterning. Small granules known as blepharoplasts are present in normal ependyma and in the well-differentiated ependymomas. These PTAH-stained gran-ules are present in the normal cell at the place where the cilia arise and in the tumour cell where the fibrillary processes are attached.

In the papillary type of ependymoma the tumour is built up of fronds or papilli with central connective tissue and blood vessels around which one or more layers of ependyma are disposed. The ependymal tumours cells may be cuboidal or columnar with their processes directed centrally into the core of the papillus. These papillary type tumours are common in the filum terminale. The epithelial type of ependymoma is the rarest but in its most typical form is the most distinctive. The tumour is made up of irregular tubules of varying sizes and lined by a single layer of ependyma-like cells. These tubules are the structures well known as "rosettes" and occur occasionally in all forms of ependymoma.

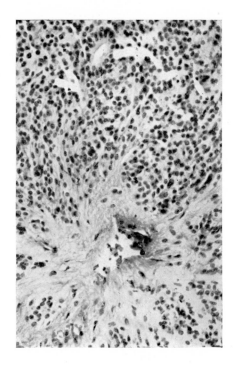

FIG. 64.—Photomicrograph of a spinal cord ependymoma. Note a "rosette" in the upper part of the picture and the perivascular orientation of the processes of the tumour cells in the lower half of the picture. Haematoxylin and eosin × 200.

They suggest a well differentiated tumour for these cells orientate themselves around a central lumen in the manner of normal ependyma in the region of the central canal.

Oligodendroglioma

These tumours are rare in the spinal cord. Slooff *et al.* (1964) had personal experience of eight cases and knew of only six other reported cases. In their clinical behaviour they resemble oligodendroglioma of the cerebrum in being slowly growing, often encapsulated tumours which, when removed, have a good prognosis except in a few instances.

Macroscopically they are not distinguishable from other intramedullary tumours. The microscopical structure is that seen in the cerebrum. The tumour architecture is that of closely packed small round or polygonal cells with very distinctive cell outlines giving a honeycomb appearance. The nuclei are equally distinct with dark chromatin content; uniformity of nuclei is a characteristic feature. The vessels of the tumour may show endothelial proliferation but necrosis and calcification have not been observed.

Mixed Gliomas and Subependymal Gliomas

As in the cerebrum an occasional glioma of the spinal cord defies classification because more than one tumour component is present. Slooff *et al.* (1964) described three such cases, two in which ependymoma was mixed with oligodendroglioma and one in which astrocytoma was mixed with oligodendroblastoma.

The problem of subependymal gliomas is rather different from that of mixed gliomas for, instead of having a mixture of two distinct types of tumour, we have a tumour of one type which is of indeterminate derivation. The tumour structure has features of astrocytoma and ependymoma and most resembles the type of glia seen normally around the ependyma of the central canal. Such tumours have been reported in the spinal cord but their true incidence is probably masked by the tendency to diagnose them either as astrocytoma or ependymoma.

Neuroblastoma, Ganglioneuroma and Ganglioglioma (Fig. 65)

I have not encountered a report of neuroblastoma of the spinal cord, but it must be remembered that the caudal dissemination of a cerebellar medulloblastoma is a common event in these tumours. There are reports of primary ganglioneuromas in the spinal cord by Kernohan *et al.* (1932), and by Lichtenstein and Zeitlin (1937). These tumours may not be separable from gangliogliomas, in which the glial stroma equals the neuronal component and like this appears neoplastic. Macroscopically these cases have small firm, circumscribed expansions of the cord. On cut section the tumour may be cystic and is frequently calcified. The microscopical appearances are those of collections of neurone-like tumour cells so disposed as to convince the observer of their neoplastic nature. Bizarre giant and deformed processes are present and the cells may be multinucleated, but mitotic figures are not seen. Calcospherites are present in the blood vessels within and sometimes around the tumour. These tumours are benign and are very slowly growing, but in their behaviour their nature is neoplastic rather than hamartomatous.

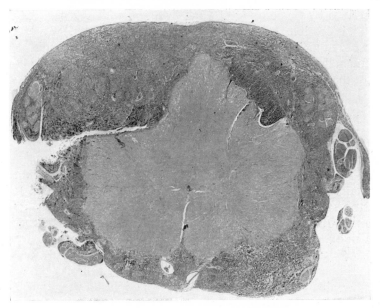

FIG. 65.—Transverse section of the spinal cord, at L1 segmental level, from a case of cerebral glioblastoma multiforme. The tumour has seeded into the subarachnoid space and surrounded the whole of the spinal cord. Haematoxylin and eosin ×7.

Teratomas, Dermoid, Epidermoid and Ependymal Cysts

These tumours and cysts are alike in being of developmental origin but only the teratoma is a true tumour. They may all occasionally be present in the spinal cord but also may occur in the spinal canal and often are associated with other developmetal anomalies.

Teratoma.—A teratoma (Willis, 1962) is a true tumour or neoplasm composed of multiple tissues of kinds foreign to the part in which it arises. In its morphology and behaviour it is distinct from such non-neoplastic malformations as parasitic twins and development cysts. Neither the spinal cord nor the spinal canal is a common site of teratoma and Willis (1960) found none in this location when studying 82 cases of teratoma. In a survey of the literature Furtado and Marques (1951) considered that approximately 20 cases of spinal teratoma had been reported of which several, all in children, had been reported by Ingraham and Bailey (1946). Subsequently there have been cases described by Cameron (1957) and by Slooff *et al.* (1964) (2 cases) and it is possible that the case of Knight *et al.* (1954–55) was of this nature. In these various case reports, tumours have occurred at all segmental levels, but rather fewer have involved the thoracic cord than the cervical cord and the lumbosacral enlargement. Associated developmental abnormalities have been common and spina bifida was present in many of the cases.

The macroscopical appearance of these tumours is very varied but usually there is a cyst, whose wall is grey or white in colour, and contains a turbid fluid, which may be mucinous or caseous. The microscopical characteristics are bizarre for these tumours contain various tissues and structures in complete disorder. It is customary to search for tissue derived from each of the three germinal layers. Ectodermally derived elements may include skin, squamous epithelium, keratin masses, hair, sweat glands, and sebaceous glands. Nervous structures may be present, usually amorphous masses of neuroglia, but sometimes neurones either of indeterminate type of suggestive of a peripheral ganglion. The various mesodermal structures are made up of bone, cartilage and muscle whilst intestinal mucosa is the common tissue present which is derived from entoderm. Various embryonal tissues may be present and these often determine the malignancy of the tumour.

Dermoid and epidermoid cysts.—These developmental cysts are clearly distinguished by Willis (1960) from teratomas, but other authors (List, 1941; Ingraham and Bailey, 1946; Rand and Rand, 1960) are doubtful whether the separation is possible or even valid in every case. Some cases, which cause taxonomic difficulty, are teratomas in which a skin-lined cavity has enlarged and dominated the tumour, giving the appearance of a dermoid or epidermoid cyst. It is doubtful whether the distinction between dermoid and epidermoid cysts, based on the histological structure of the cyst wall, can be held, for in their origin and behaviour they appear identical. These cysts are commoner than teratomas and there have been several full acounts which have discussed intraspinal cases. An early case was reported by Chiari (1883) and concerned a 33-year-old man who had an intramedullary epidermoid at T4–6 spinal cord level. Good reviews of cases are present in the reports of List (1941), Sachs and Horrax (1949), Tytus and Pennybacker (1956), Rand and Rand (1960) and Manno *et al.* (1962). In some cases (Boyd, 1966) there is evidence that an epidermoid cyst is iatrogenic, being derived from tissue implanted during lumbar puncture.

Dermoid and epidermoid cysts are found at all levels of the spinal canal but are commoner in its lower portion. They may be wholly intramedullary, wholly extramedullary or may be partly inside and partly outside the spinal cord. In their most typical form they present as an expansion of the cauda equina, often become very large, and fill the lower part of the spinal canal. X-radiographs may show widening of the interpeduncular space or erosion of the pedicles and the posterior surfaces of the vertebral bodies. Associated abnormalities of development are common, the most constant being spina bifida. Several reported cases have had dermal sinuses extending through a spina bifida into a sub-cutaneous mass. The histological structure of the wall of these cysts is variable but the constant feature is a lining of squamous epithelium. Skin appendages such as hair, and sebaceous and sweat glands may be present in the connective tissue outside the inner squamous layer. The cysts are filled with the products of these structures, mainly keratin but sometimes hair and sebum. Other cystic structures affecting the spinal cord are dealt with in Chapter II and arachnoid cysts are described with adhesive spinal arachnoiditis in Chapter VIII.

Other Intramedullary Tumours

The remaining intramedullary tumours are all rare. It would be expected that the supporting vascular and connective tissue of the spinal cord would occasionally be the origin of neoplasms and a few tumours of this nature have been reported. Slooff *et al.* (1964) described a malignant fibrosarcoma of the filum terminale in a man of 40 years. These authors also reported two cases of schwann-oma arising in the spinal cord, presumably from perivascular nerves accompanying spinal arteries. In a review of the literature of intramedullary schwannomas, they could find only the single cases reported by Riggs and Clary (1957), Ramamurthi *et al.* (1958), and Scott and Bentz (1962). There are several recorded cases of haemangioblastoma of the spinal cord, a condition reviewed by Krishnan and Smith (1961).

Lipomas are rare, but so curious is their intramedullary occurrence that several reviews of the subject have been made (Sperling and Alpers, 1936; Ehni and Love, 1945; Johnson, 1950; and Rogers *et al.*, 1971). The reader is referred to these papers for the controversial question of their origin. It should however be noted that in many cases the lipoma is not wholly intramedullary and that often there is an associated spina bifida. The macroscopical appearance of these tumours in this situation is not different from other intramedullary neoplasms. Histologically they are similar to lipomas in other situations; that is, made up of adult fat cells.

Secondary metastatic tumours of the spinal cord require only brief mention. They are usually considered rare but in advanced disseminated carcinomatosis may occur undetected, since the spinal cord is seldom examined in these cases. As a solitary meta-stasis the case attracts more attention from clinician and path-ologist. Willis (1952) discussed twelve case reports and Benson (1960) described three cases of intramedullary metastasis (from bronchogenic carcinoma) and reviewed 24 similar cases. There have been subsequent accounts by Chason et al. (1963) who reported ten cases and Sherbourne et al. (1964) who reported three cases. The primary tumours of these 40 cases of spinal-cord meta-stasis were made up as follows: Bronchogenic carcinoma, 22 cases, breast carcinoma, three cases; kidney carcinoma, three cases; malignant melanoma, three cases; adrenal carcinoma, one case; colonic carcinoma, one case; chorionepithelioma, one case; testicular sarcoma, one case; Hodgkins' disease, one case. In four cases (Chason et al., 1963) the source of the primary tumour was not given in the report which was a survey, based on necropsy examinations, of metastases of carcinomas to the central nervous system. They found metastatic carcinoma of the central nervous system in 200 (18.3 per cent) of 1096 patients with carcinoma. Their series provides a valuable estimate of the incidence of meta-static carcinoma in the spinal cord, since they examined this structure post-mortem in every case. Intramedullary metastases were found in 10 cases which represented an incidence of 5 per cent of their cases with central nervous system involvement and 1 per cent of all their cases of carcinoma (including malignant melanoma).

EXTRAMEDULLARY TUMOURS

A large number of primary and secondary tumours affect the spinal canal and it would be out of place here to detail all of these occurrences. In the manner in which the spinal cord is damaged the main difference is whether the tumour is a slow growing benign one or a malignant infiltrative and destructive type of tumour, either primary or secondary in origin.

Benign Tumours

The benign tumours affecting the spinal canal are all rare with the exception of the neurofibroma and the meningioma, and these tumours are very important causes of remediable cord compression.

Neurofibromas and schwannomas.—The controversy about nomenclature and the separation into two types, with the names of neurofibroma and schwannoma, of tumours of the nerve roots and peripheral nerves, has been admirably reviewed by Russell and Rubinstein (1963). With some exceptions, neurofibromas are multiple tumours of cranial and spinal nerve roots and of peripheral nerves. The syndrome includes many other developmental abnormalities and constitutes von Recklinghausen's disease of nerve (Fig. 66). The neurofibroma appears as an expansion of the nerve from which it originates, which appears to traverse the tumour. The microscopical structure is that of irregularly arranged masses of bipolar, spindle-shaped cells with tapering processes. Mitotic figures are not seen except in the rare malignant examples which have the histological appearance of a cellular fibrosarcoma.

The schwannoma is usually solitary, but multiple tumours are not very rare and some of the numerous tumours of a case

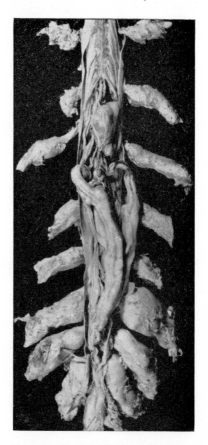

FIG. 66.—Von Recklinghausen's disease of nerve. Neurofibromata are present on every nerve root and the tumours involving the cauda equina form an interlocking mass of tumour distending the dura mater. The specimen is viewed from the anterior aspect.

of von Recklinghausen's disease may be schwannomas. The tumour is encapsulated and often appears attached to nerve rather than traversed by a nerve. The histological structure is of two types. In the type A tissue of Antoni (1920) there are interwoven bundles of spindle cells whose nuclei are often arranged in parallel rows (palisading). The type B tissue of Antoni is loose spongy tissue, probably a degenerative form of the type A tissue.

The neurofibromas and schwannomas occur in the spinal canal impartially on any of the spinal nerve roots (Elsberg, 1941). They usually have no attachment to dura and consequently are more mobile than are meningiomas. They may occasionally arise on a

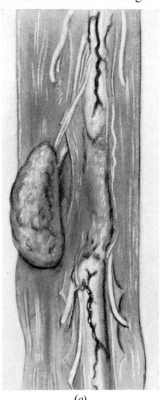

(a)

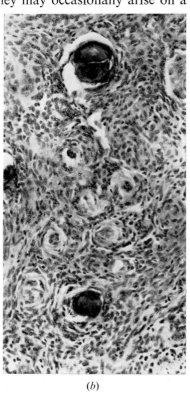

(b)

Fig. 67a.—Drawing of a post-mortem specimen of a spinal meningioma. The dura has been opened from the anterior aspect and reflected, revealing the tumour on the right side.

Fig. 67b.—Photomicrograph of a spinal meningioma. The whorl formation and the psammoma bodies are common in this type of tumour. Haematoxylin and eosin ×170.

nerve root within an intervertebral foramen and extend both into the spinal canal and out of the foramen into, for example, the thoracic cavity. From the shape of the resulting tumour mass these nerve tumours are often called dumb-bell tumours.

Meningiomas (Fig. 67a, b).—Within the theca these tumours were the commonest tumours and accounted for 24 per cent of 190 cases of spinal cord compression at the Radcliffe Infirmary, Oxford (Penny-backer, 1958). They are commoner in middle life and in women. They are attached to the inner surface of the dura, are invested by the arach-noid, have a firm capsule, and al-though they may be closely adherent to the cord they do not invade it. The thoracic region is more often involved than other levels and the tumours are frequently laterally situated. They may rarely be extradural in situation, and Calogero and Moossy (1972) re-viewed 35 cases of this type. The tumour reported by Hallpike and Stanley (1968) was an extradural meningioma which had extended into the thorax through an intervertebral foramen, thus forming a dumb-bell tumour. The histological structure of these spinal meningiomas is similar to that of the intracranial examples except that slow-growing psammo-matous types with abundant calcified concretions are more common.

Other benign tumours of the spinal canal.—All the remaining benign

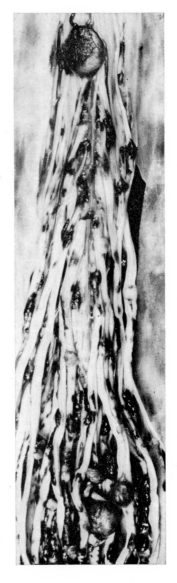

FIG. 68.—Primary malignant melanoma of the leptomeninges. The picture is of the anterior aspect of the caudal part of the spinal cord. The dura has been reflected to show the numerous melanomata growing on the spinal nerve roots.

tumours affecting the spinal canal are rare. The lipomas have already been mentioned with the intramedullary neoplasms, but they occur more frequently outside the spinal cord. Cavernous haemangioma of the vertebrae (Bailey and Bucy, 1929), which has a very characteristic roentgenological picture, is a rare cause of cord compression and so are the following tumours: Osteoblastoma (osteoid fibroma), Rand and Rand (1960); osteoclastoma, Jaffe (1958); osteoid osteoma, Sherman (1947), Sabanas *et al.* (1956), and Heilbrun and Lehman (1971).

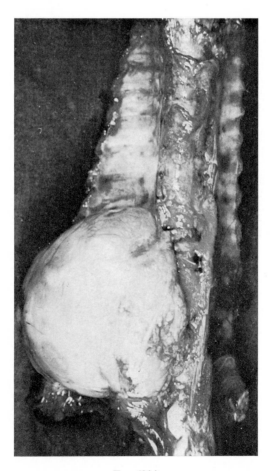

Fig. 69(*a*)

Malignant Tumours

The malignant extramedullary tumours which affect the spinal cord are of varying tissue origin but the commonest by far are the secondary metastases of various carcinomas. Barron *et al.* (1959) in analysing 127 necropsied cases of these tumours found the various types occurred in the following order of frequency: Bronchogenic carcinoma, breast carcinoma, lymphoma, renal carcinoma, myeloma, sarcoma, prostatic carcinoma, rectal carcinoma, uterine carcinoma, thyroid carcinoma. There were, in this series, single cases of hepatoma, ovarian carcinoma, lymphoepithelioma of the nasopharynx, malignant mixed parotid tumour, seminoma, pancreatic carcinoma and malignant melanoma. From my own experience I would add neuroblastoma and haemangio-endothelioma to this list. The lymphomas are an important group in these cases and instances of Hodgkin's

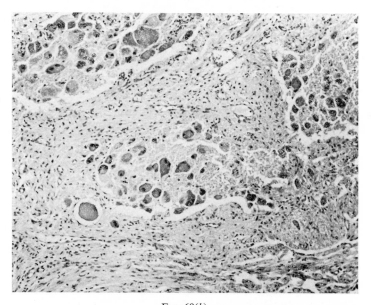

Fig. 69(*b*)

Fig. 69.—Ganglioneuroma. (*a*) A large spherical tumour, arising from the thoracic sympathetic ganglia, has spread via the right T10 and T11 intervertebral foramina into the spinal canal. The spinal cord was encircled by tumour and compressed. (*b*) Photomicrograph of tumour within the spinal canal. There are islands of tumour cells resembling adult neuronal cell bodies and these are embedded in a matrix made up chiefly of cell processes. Haematoxylin and eosin ×120.

disease, lymphosarcoma, reticulosarcoma, and the leukaemias are all regularly seen in a busy neurosurgical service.

Primary melanoma of the leptomeninges is a rare tumour presenting usually as multiple disseminated malignant growths (Fig. 68). Figure 69a, b shows a ganglioneuroma which had spread into the spinal canal via an intervertebral foramen.

In the common forms of malignant paraplegia the mechanism by which the spinal cord is damaged varies from case to case and when a large series of necropsied cases is analysed the type of damage falls into one or more of four categories.

I. **Vertebral collapse.**—When the vertebral bodies are the seat of a primary malignant tumour such as a myeloma, a chordoma

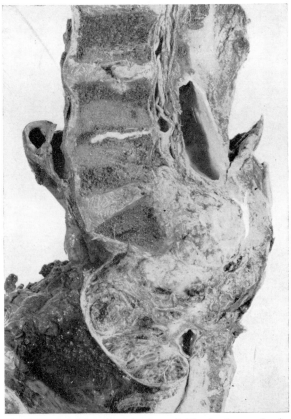

FIG. 70.—Chordoma involving the spinal canal. The lumbosacral spine has been sawn sagittally to show the involvement of the spinal canal by a chordoma. Note the destruction and replacement of the sacrum by tumour.

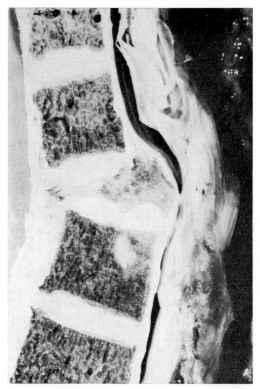

FIG. 71.—Malignant paraplegia from carcinoma of the bronchus. The spine had been sawn sagittally to show the spinal cord within the spinal canal. There is angulation at T2 body which has collapsed due to infiltration by metastatic tumour also seen in T3 body.

(Fig. 70) or a secondary malignant tumour (Fig. 71) the erosion of bone causes collapse of one or more vertebrae. This collapse, which may be rapid in onset, results in angulation of the spinal canal with compression of the spinal cord against a spur of the hinged canal. The damage to the spinal cord is similar to that in Pott's paraplegia and in osteoporosis.

II. **Malignant infiltration within the canal.**—This type of spread occurs in carcinomas, but is particularly common in the malignant tumours of the reticulo-endothelial system. In these tumours, the growth is more infiltrative and there is usually considerable tumour in the extradural space which may compress the cord. Invasion of the intradural space is also common and seems particularly likely in the leukaemias.

III. **Spinal-cord infarction.**—When, in a case of widespread malignant tumour, there is tumour completely surrounding the spinal column, it is possible that, by obliteration of its radicular tributaries in the intervertebral foramina, the spinal cord is infarcted. I have seen this complication in several cases of carcinomatosis, in reticulosis and in malignant haemangio-endothelioma.

IV. **Intramedullary metastasis.**—This is the fourth and rarest type, which has been described earlier.

REFERENCES

ANTONI, N. (1920). *Ueber Rückenmarkstumoren und Neurofibrome.* Munich: Bergmann.

BAILEY, P. and BUCY, P. C. (1929). Cavernous hemangioma of the vertebrae. *J. Amer. med. Ass.*, **92**, 1748–1751.

BAILEY, P. and CUSHING, H. (1926). *A Classification of the Tumours of the Glioma Group on a Histogenetic Basis with a Correlated Study of Prognosis.* Philadelphia: Lippincott.

BARRON, K. D., HIRANO, A., ARAKI, S. and TERRY, R. D. (1959). Experiences with metastatic neoplasms involving the spinal cord. *Neurology (Minneap.)*, **9**, 91–106.

BENSON, D. F. (1960). Intramedullary spinal cord metastasis. *Neurology (Minneap.)*, **10**, 281–287.

BOYD, H. R. (1966). Iatrogenic intraspinal epidermoid. *J. Neurosurg.*, **24**, 105–107.

CALOGERO, J. A. and MOOSSY, J. (1972). Extradural spinal meningiomas. Report of four cases. *J. Neurosurg.*, **37**, 442–447.

CAMERON, A. H. (1957). Malformations of the neuro-spinal axis, urogenital tract and foregut in spina bifida attributable to disturbances of the blastopore. *J. Path. Bact.*, **73**, 213–221.

CHASON, J. L., WALKER, F. B. and LANDERS, J. W. (1963). Metastatic carcinoma in the central nervous system and dorsal root ganglia. *Cancer (Philad.)*, **16**, 781–787.

CHIARI, H. (1883). Centrales Cholesteatoma des Dorsalmarkes mit vollkommen entrickelter auf- und absteigender Degeneration. *Prag. med. Wschr.*, **39**, 378–380.

CRUVEILHIER, J. (1835–42). *Anatomie pathologique du corps humain.* Paris: Baillière.

EHNI, G. and LOVE, J. G. (1945). Intraspinal lipomas; report of cases; review of the literature, and clinical and pathologic study. *Arch. Neurol. Psychiat. (Chic.)*, **53**, 1–28.

ELSBERG, C. A. (1941). *Surgical Diseases of the Spinal Cord, Membranes, and Nerve Roots.* New York: Hoeber.

FURTADO, D. and MARQUES, V. (1951). Spinal teratoma. *J. Neuropath. exp. Neurol.*, **10**, 384–393.

GOWERS, W. R. and HORSLEY, V. A. (1888). A case of tumour of the spinal cord; removal: recovery. *Med.-chir. Trans.*, **71**, 377–430.

HALLPIKE, J. F. and STANLEY, P. (1968). A case of extradural spinal meningioma. *J. Neurol. Neurosurg. Psychiat.*, **31**, 195–197.

HEILBRUN, M. P. and LEHMAN, R. A. W. (1971). Osteoid osteoma of the cervical spine. *J. Neurosurg.*, **35**, 331–334.

HENSCHEN, F. (1955). Tumoren des Zentralnervensystems und seiner Hüllen. In *Handbuch der Speziellen Pathologischen Anatomie und Histologie*, Vol. XIII/3, pp. 413–1040. Ed. by W. Scholz. Berlin-Göttingen-Heidelberg: Springer.

INGRAHAM, F. D. and BAILEY, O. T. (1946). Cystic teratomas and teratoid tumours of the central nervous system in infancy and childhood. *J. Neurosurg.*, **3**, 511–532.

JAFFE, H. L. (1958). *Tumours and Tumorous Conditions of the Bones and Joints*. London: Kimpton.

JOHNSON, D. F. (1950). Intramedullary lipoma of the spinal cord, review of the literature and report of case. *Bull. Los Angeles neurol. Soc.*, **15**, 37–42.

KERNOHAN, J. W., LEARMONTH, J. R. and DOYLE, J. B. (1932). Neuroblastomas and gangliocytomas of central nervous system. *Brain*, **55**, 287–310.

KERNOHAN, J. W. and SAYRE, G. P. (1952). Tumours of the central nervous system. In *Atlas of Tumour Pathology*, Section X, Fasc. 35 and 37. Washington: Armed Forces Institute of Pathology.

KNIGHT, G., GRIFFITHS, T. and WILLIAMS, I. (1954–55). Gastrocystoma of the spinal cord. *Brit. J. Surg.*, **42**, 635–638.

KRISHNAN, K. R. and SMITH, W. T. (1961). Intramedullary haemangioblastoma of the spinal cord associated with pial varicosities simulating intradural angioma. *J. Neurol. Neurosurg. Psychiat.*, **24**, 350–352.

LICHTENSTEIN, B. W. and ZEITLIN, H. (1937). Ganglioneuroma of spinal cord associated with pseudosyringomyelia. Histologic study. *Arch. Neurol. Psychiat. (Chic.)*, **37**, 1356–1370.

LIST, C. F. (1941). Intraspinal epidermoids, dermoids, and dermal sinuses. *Surg. Gynec. Obstet.*, **73**, 525–538.

MABON, R. F., SVIEN, H. J., KERNOHAN, J. W. and CRAIG, W. M. (1949). Ependymomas. *Proc. Mayo Clin.*, **24**, 65–71.

MANNO, N. J., UIHLEIN, A. and KERNOHAN, J. W. (1962). Intraspinal epidermoids. *J. Neurosurg.*, **19**, 754–765.

MORGAGNI, G. B. (1761). *De Sedibus et Causis Morborum*, Book 1, II, act 23.

OLLIVIER, C. P. (1837). *Traité des maladies de la moelle épinière*, 3rd. edit. Paris: Méquignon-Marvis.

PENNYBACKER, J. (1958). Malignant tumours of the brain, spinal cord, and peripheral nerves. In *Cancer*, Vol. 4, Ed. by R. W. Raven. London: Butterworth.

PHILLIPS, T. (1792). An account of a tumour situated in the lumbar vertebrae of a very extraordinary size and singular appearance and which ensued from a fall. *New London med. J.*, **1**, 144–148.

RAMAMURTHI, B., ANGULI, V. C. and IYER, C. G. S. (1958). A case of intramedullary neurinoma. *J. Neurol. Neurosurg. Psychiat.*, **21**, 92–94.

RAND, R. W. and RAND, C. W. (1960). *Intraspinal Tumours of Childhood*. Springfield, Ill.: Charles Thomas.

RIGGS, H. E. and CLARY, W. U. (1957). A case of intramedullary sheath cell tumour of the spinal cord: consideration of vascular nerves as a source of origin. *J. Neuropath. exp. Neurol.*, **16**, 332–336.

ROGERS, H. M., LONG, D. M., CHOU, S. N. and FRENCH, L. A. (1971). Lipomas of the spinal cord and cauda equina. *J. Neurosurg.*, **34**, 349–354.

RUSSELL, D. S. and RUBINSTEIN, L. J. (1971). *Pathology of Tumours of the Nervous System*. 3rd edit. London: Edward Arnold.

SABANAS, A. O., BICKEL, W. H. and MOE, J. H. (1956). Natural history of osteoid osteoma of the spine; review of the literature and report of three cases. *Amer. J. Surg.*, **91**, 880–889.

SACHS, E. and HORRAX, G. (1949). A cervical and a lumbar pilonidal sinus communicating with intraspinal dermoids. *J. Neurosurg.*, **6**, 97–112.

SCOTT, M. and BENTZ, R. (1962). Intramedullary neurilemmoma (neurinoma) of the thoracic cord. A case report. *J. Neuropath. exp. Neurol.*, **21**, 194–200.

SHERBOURNE, D. H., TRIBE, C. R. and VARMA, S. (1964). Intramedullary spinal cord metastases. A clinico-pathological report of three cases. *Int. J. Paraplegia*, **2**, 100–111.

SHERMAN, M. S. (1947). Osteoid osteoma; review of the literature and report of thirty cases. *J. Bone Jt Surg.*, **29A**, 918–930.

SLOOFF, J. L., KERNOHAN, J. W. and MACCARTY, C. S. (1964). *Primary Intramedullary Tumours of the Spinal Cord and Filum Terminale*, Philadelphia: Saunders.

SPERLING, S. J. and ALPERS, B. J. (1936). Lipoma and osteolipoma of the brain. *J. nerv. ment. Dis.*, **83**, 13–21.

TARLOV, I. M. (1957). *Spinal Cord Compression. Mechanisms of Paralysis and Treatment*. Springfield, Ill.: Charles Thomas.

TARLOV, I. M. (1972). Acute spinal cord compression paralysis. *J. Neurosurg.*, **36**, 10–20.

TYTUS, J. S. and PENNYBACKER, J. (1956). Pearly tumours in relation to the central nervous system. *J. Neurol. Neurosurg. Psychiat.*, **19**, 241–259.

WILLIS, R. A. (1952). *The Spread of Tumours in the Human Body*. 2nd edit., London: Butterworth.

WILLIS, R. A. (1960). *Pathology of Tumours*. 3rd edit. London: Butterworth.

WILLIS, R. A. (1962). *The Borderland of Embryology and Pathology*. 2nd edit. London: Butterworth.

CHAPTER XI

NECROPSY EXAMINATION
OF THE SPINAL CORD

The spinal column, such a flexible yet strong protection for its contents, poses a barrier to those inexperienced in the necropsy examination of the spinal cord. As I am frequently asked to advise on methods of removing an examining the spinal cord, I have gathered here some of the details that make the difference between success and failure.

Clinical Information of the Case

I do not think it superfluous to remind the pathologist of the importance of informing himself of all clinical details relevant to the case. The nerve plexuses, motor and cutaneous nerves, autonomic nerves, skin, and voluntary muscles form such a wealth of material that even a reasonably comprehensive histological examination can only be a small sample of the total tissue in which the disease may be manifest. For this reason it is essential that the sample should be taken wisely and this can only be done in relation to the clinical details available.

The General Necropsy

A neuropathologist must also be a competent general morbid anatomist. It is idle to examine the spinal cord without reference to the other necropsy findings, which should be carefully sought, considered and recorded in full. The situation and extent of tumours, particularly primary or secondary around the spine should be noted in detail. The adequacy of the blood supply to the spinal cord may prove to be important and for this reason a record of the state of the aorta, and of the vertebral, intercostal and lumbar arteries is essential. Equally important may be the state of the venous drainage of the spinal cord. These factors are difficult to evaluate after the necropsy and conjecture is no substitute for fact. In certain cases injection of the spinal cord blood supply with a suitable contrast material, before, at, or after the necropsy may be desirable. This may be simply performed by injecting relevant arteries, such as the vertebral arteries, intercostal arteries *etc.* (see Chapter IV), with a suitable injection fluid introduced by a 10 or 20 ml syringe. Indian ink may be used but there are advantages (and difficulties) in using Neoprene latex (B.B. Chemical Co. Ltd., Leicester, England) or Marco resin (Scott Bader and Co. Ltd., 109 Kingsway, London, W.C.2). For information about injection techniques, the account of Tompsett (1956) will be found invaluable.

For two reasons, the removal of the spine with the spinal cord *in situ* is to be preferred. The unfixed spinal cord is easily damaged *post-mortem* whilst the fixed cord can be safely handled. Secondly in the spinal specimen we have spinal nerve roots, posterior root ganglia and most of the spinal cord blood supply, all of which may subsequently prove important in an understanding of the case. If this recommended procedure cannot be followed and the spinal cord must be removed in the necropsy room, then the cadaver should be placed in the prone position and the operator should follow the instructions in "Removal of the spinal cord from the spine".

Removal of the Spine (Fig. 72*a*, *b*, *c*)

The body is left in the supine position after the general autopsy has been carried out. Remove the brain, cutting through the lower medulla as transversely as possible. With a strong scalpel cut through the dura in a circle around the foramen magnum, inserting the scalpel deeply to sever the connections between the atlas and the occipital condyles. Now, with a small handsaw, make two oblique cuts through the sacrum near the sacroiliac joints, the cuts meeting posteriorly and freeing the sacrum and spine from the pelvic girdle. The lower end of the spine can now be lifted up, whilst with a scalpel the soft tissues are detached, proceeding upwards until the thoracic cage is reached. Then saw through each rib as near to the spine as possible, in this way making the spine loose and held only by soft tissues which may be detached with a scalpel. There now remains only the task of detaching the spine from the occipital condyles, completing the task begun from above. This procedure, although appearing formidable, is rapidly accomplished and 10–15 minutes usually suffices. The body is reconstituted with wood; a broomstick is convenient, the sharpened lower end being thrust into the remains of the sacrum, whilst the upper end is inserted through the foramen magnum.

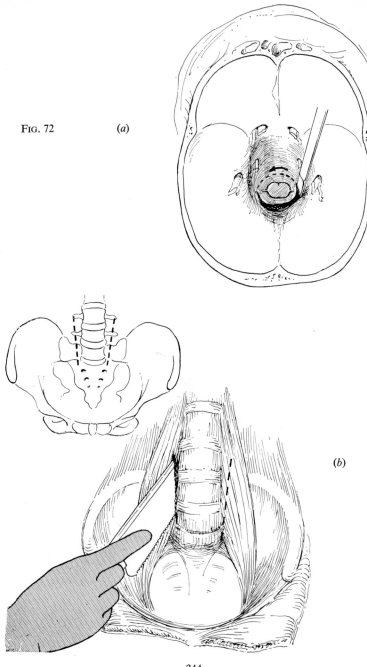

FIG. 72 (*a*)

(*b*)

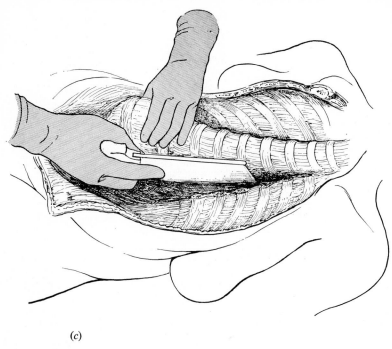

(*c*)

FIG. 72.—Removal of the spine at necropsy.
   (*a*) Cutting through the dura and separating the atlas vertebra from the occipital condyles.
   (*b*) Freeing the sacrum from the pelvis by two oblique saw cuts. The small diagram shows the position of these cuts in relation to the bony pelvis.
   (*c*) Mobilising the spine by sawing through the ribs.

Finally a crosspiece of wood is placed across the shoulders and all the woodframe covered with cotton waste or plaster of Paris.

Correctly carried out this procedure should cause no added disfigurement to that of a conventional necropsy.

Removal of the Spinal Cord from the Spine (Fig. 73*a*, *b*, *c*)

This should be undertaken after fixation in formalin for one to three weeks. The fixed spine is secured in a vice, the posterior aspect upwards. Most of the spinal musculature is now removed allowing the spinal laminae to be seen. With either a small hand saw or an electric saw (necropsy saw Type NS 2000, Desoutter Bros. Ltd. London), the laminae are sawn through. The position and angle of the saw cut is most important (see diagram), and

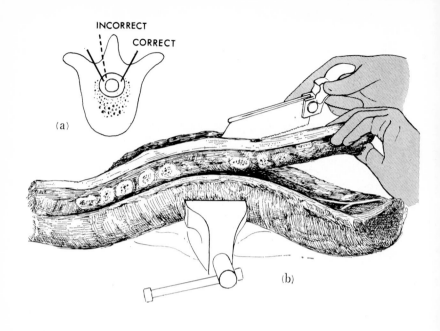

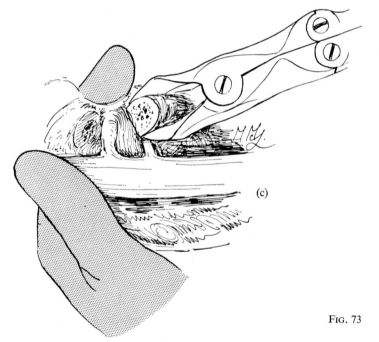

INCORRECT
CORRECT

(a)

(b)

(c)

Fig. 73

246

incorrect laminectomy is the commonest serious error made. After removal of the laminae, a little extradural fat is cleared away to expose the dura throughout the whole length of the spinal cord. The caudal end of the dural sac is now gripped in an artery forceps, in order that one may gently raise the cord whilst, with a scalpel or sharp scissors, each root is cut, working upwards from below. If it is desired to have the roots and posterior ganglia attached to the cord, these can be exposed by nibbling away the posterior walls of the intervertebral foramina, working always laterally outwards from the cord. The dural sheaths should first be identified and the tips of the forceps follow the dural tube into the foramen. For this work strong bone forceps are required and I have always preferred Swedish pattern laminectomy shears.

Identification of Spinal Cord Segments

Contrary to the opinion of some, the expert neuropathologist cannot identify with certainty any given spinal cord segment either macroscopically or in a stained section. The anatomical peculiarities of a segment that may allow its recognition may be obscured by disease and even in the normal cord many of the thoracic segments cannot be distinguished from one another. However, by following the procedure given here, even the inexpert can identify all the segments of the spinal cord.

The first step is to identify T1 which of all the segments is the most distinctive. At this point the flattened cervical enlargement gives way to the thoracic cord which is round in cross section. The roots of T2 (anterior and posterior) are of equal size as are all the subsequent thoracic nerve roots. The roots of T1 are unequal, the posterior root being larger than the anterior. Both are larger than the roots of T2. The cervical roots have several distinctive features but the most reliable is that C5, 6, 7 and 8 anterior roots are large whilst the upper four cervical roots are small. Note that you may not find or notice the small C1 roots. A transverse cut or cuts through T1 will confirm its identification. The grey matter of C8 has the typical configuration of a cervical segment whilst T2

Fig. 73 (*see opposite*).—Removal of the spinal cord from the spine.

(*a*) Diagram showing position and direction of the saw cuts through the vertebral laminae.

(*b*) Removing the spinous processes and laminae and exposing the spinal canal from behind.

(*c*) Exposing the intervertebral foramina with bone forceps.

has grey matter typical of a thoracic segment (lateral horn *etc.*). The T1 segment is the region of change, its upper part being like a cervical segment, whilst its lower part is like T2. If one is still in doubt then recourse to the spine will settle any lingering uncertainty. In the spine the vertebral bodies can be readily identified (a sagittal saw cut is helpful), then the spinal nerve roots can be seen passing into their foramina. Note that T1 nerve root passes into a foramen beneath T1 vertebra and such correspondence is regular throughout the thoracic and lower spine. The cervical region is of course different; C8 root emerges below C7 vertebra *etc*. The L1 nerve roots can often be recognised by a feature of the dentate ligament that is at times helpful. The dentate ligament, which is formed by regular attachments of the pia-arachnoid to the lateral meninges, ends by a distinct fork, the lateral part being a strong slip going to an attachment to the lateral meninges, whilst the medial part of the fork blends with the pia-arachnoid passing caudally to form eventually the filum terminale. This fork of the dentate ligament is helpful in that the L1 nerve root normally lies upon it. This is a useful check on the identification based on the T1 segment. Having found the T1 and L1 segments, all others can be identified by counting up and down.

Preparation of Histological Sections (Fig. 74)

Whilst longitudinal sections are occasionally useful the most informative sections from the spinal cord are those cut in the transverse plane. The number of transverse sections required is dependent on the nature and position of the lesion. However even if one block of tissue is taken from each spinal-cord segment (31 in all) this should not be too laborious if the following procedure is carried out. Blocks of approximately 0.5 cm are cut from each segment and are placed caudal surface uppermost on a sheet of paper. When the surface has been dried with filterpaper, the name of the segment can be written on the actual tissue using a camel hair brush and a waterproof type ink. When this is dry all the blocks may be processed together in a single container in which they are dehydrated and cleared. They are sorted just before the embedding process. From 5 to 10 blocks of tissue can be embedded and cut together, the number being determined by the dexterity of one's histology technician. I have always preferred embedding in paraffin wax and consider the celloidin techniques to be unnecessary in examining the spinal cord. It is not necessary to give details here of staining procedures since many excellent accounts exist (Anderson, 1929; Carleton, 1957; Gasser, 1961). The book by Ráliš *et al.* (1973) contains all the methods in regular use in the author's laboratory. It is important to perfect a good myelin stain (Weil, Loyez or similar) but otherwise the familiar haematoxylin and eosin, and haematoxylin and Van Gieson of general morbid anatomy will be found the most valuable. It might reassure newcomers to neuropathology to learn that, in a case of

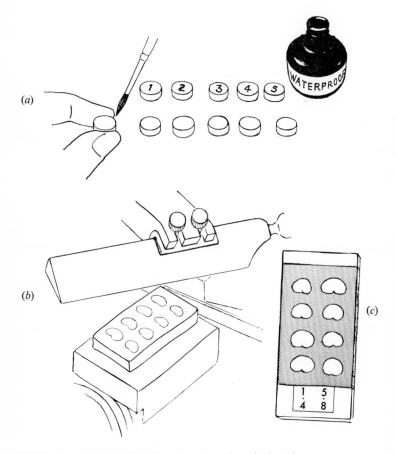

FIG. 74.—Preparing histological sections from the spinal cord.
  (*a*) Marking transversely cut blocks of spinal cord with waterproof carbon ink.
  (*b*) Cutting a paraffin block in which multiple segments of spinal cord are embedded.
  (*c*) Stained slide with eight sections of the spinal cord prepared simultaneously.

spinal-cord disease, about 90 per cent of the information may be gleaned from these three stains. It is traditional to examine neurone cell bodies in Nissl-stained sections, but most of the observations may be made with the haematoxylin and eosin stain. The purpose of these remarks is to encourage those un-familiar with specialised neuropathological techniques, which it is not my intention to decry. Indeed, I feel deeply grateful for the range of elegant staining techniques available in the nervous system, some of which impart not only factual information but aesthetic pleasure. Two stains, both applicable to paraffin-embedded sections, are especially valuable, although technically difficult for the inexpert. Holzer's method for glial fibres is the most convenient way of demonstrating astrocytic fibrous gliosis and Holmes' stain gives excellent staining of nerve axons both in the spinal cord and in its nerve roots.

Microscopical Examination of the Spinal Cord

In this work, a binocular low-power microscope is almost indispensable, otherwise one must rely on a good hand lens. This emphasis on critical low-power observation also obtains in the compound microscope for which good low-power objectives and an appropriate condenser system should be sought.

(i) **Meninges and vessels.**—These are examined in the haema-toxylin and eosin and in the haematoxylin and Van Gieson stains. It is difficult to evaluate connective tissue thickening of the leptomeninges which may be the result of a former pyogenic meningitis, a toxic irritant in the subarachnoid space, or meningo-vascular syphilis. The difficulty is that moderate leptomeningeal thickening is a common finding in an elderly spinal cord and other evidence of its significance must be sought, and may be found in an inspection of the vessels. Atheroma is extremely rare in the vessels of the spinal cord but may affect the spinal cord by involve-ment of the aorta and other major arteries. In these circumstances the small intramedullary vessels may show changes suggestive of chronic ischaemia.

(ii) **Grey matter.**—Absence or depletion of neurones is looked for in the Nissl or haematoxylin and eosin stains and the gliosis evoked by long-standing cell loss may be seen in the Holzer stain. In these observations a knowledge of the normal population and the structure of the grey matter is essential and the atlases of Bruce (1901) and Riley (1943) are recommended. The neurone cell bodies may show significant reactive changes and for a description of axonal reaction and ischaemic changes the reader is referred to Chapter I.

(iii) **White matter.**—Here the myelin stains (Weil or Loyez) are essential, but useful information may be derived from the haematoxylin and Van Gieson stain. Long-tract degeneration is looked for particularly in the posterior columns (gracile and cuneate tracts) and the lateral columns (corticospinal tracts). Note that immediately above or below a spinal cord lesion the fibre degeneration is rather diffuse and indistinct. Further caudal or cephalad the Wallerian degeneration becomes more apparent because the fibres of the long tracts move more closely together in their bundles.

(iv) **Spinal nerve roots.**—These may usually be inspected in the myelin and in the Holmes' stains of the transverse sections of the spinal cord. The orientation of the nerve fibres may not be appropriate and in certain cases special blocks may be taken of nerve roots and of posterior root ganglia. It is a feature of most myelin stains that the portion of nerve root immediately outside the spinal cord stains badly. This should not be mistaken for root atrophy which can be checked by the finding of axon depletion in the Holmes' stain.

(v) **Correlation of clinical and pathological findings.**—The final solution of a case of this nature includes the correct explanation of the clinical findings by the pathological findings. In a retrospective consideration of the clinical history, take particular and detailed note of disturbances of sensation and of paralysis affecting limbs, trunk, bladder and bowel. Do not accept uncritically dubious clinical evidence of sensory disturbance or even weakness, for this may be the weakness of prostration and have no demonstrable basis in the nervous system. Look for clinical evidence of muscle wasting, for this, if described precisely, gives an accurate localisation in the spinal cord of the lesion, which, in my experience, will invariably be found.

REFERENCES

ANDERSON, J. (1929). *How to Stain the Nervous System*. Edinburgh: Livingstone.

BRUCE, A. (1901). *A Topographical Atlas of the Spinal Cord*. Edinburgh: Williams and Norgate.

CARLETON, H. M. (1957). *Histological Technique*, 3rd edit. London: Oxford University Press.

GASSER, G. (1961). *Basic Neuropathological Technique*. Oxford: Blackwell Scientific Publications.

RÁLIŠ, H. M., BEESLEY, R. A. and RÁLIŠ, Z. A. (1973). *Techniques in Neurohistology*. London: Butterworth.

RILEY, H. A. (1943). *An Atlas of the Basal Ganglia, Brain Stem and Spinal Cord*. Baltimore: Williams and Wilkins.

TOMPSETT, D. H. (1956). *Anatomical Techniques*. Edinburgh: Livingstone.

GENERAL REFERENCES

The author recommends the following books for general reference:

BLACKWOOD, W. (1976). (Editor.) *Greenfield's Neuropathology*, 3rd edit. London: Edward Arnold.

BOURNE, G. H. (1968–72). (Editor.) *The Structure and Function of Nervous Tissues*, Vols. 1–6. New York: Academic Press.

CAJAL, S. RAMÓN (1952). *Histologie du systeme nerveux de l'homme et des vertébrés*, Vols. 1 and 2. Madrid: Instituto Ramón y Cajal.

CAJAL, S. RAMÓN (1959). *Degeneration and Regeneration of the Nervous System*, Vols. 1 and 2. New York: Hafner.

LUBARSCH, O., HENKE, F. and RÖSSLE, R. (1955–58). *Handbuch der Speziellen Pathologischen Anatomie und Histologie*, Vol. XIII. Ed. by W. Scholz. Berlin-Göttingen-Heidelberg: Springer.

MINCKLER, J. (1968–72). (Editor.) *Pathology of the Nervous System*, Vols. 1–3. New York: McGraw-Hill.

PENFIELD, W. (1932). (Editor.) *Cytology and Cellular Pathology of the Nervous System*. Vols. 1–3. New York: Hoeber.

RUBINSTEIN, L. J. (1972). *Tumours of the Central Nervous System* (2nd Series, Fasc. 6. Atlas of Tumor Pathology.) Washington, D.C.: Armed Forces Institute of Pathology.

RUSSELL, D. S. and RUBINSTEIN, L. J. (1971). *Pathology of Tumours of the Nervous System*, 3rd edit. London: Edward Arnold.

INDEX